W9-CPB-837

Working Safe

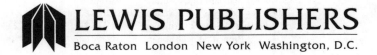

How to Help People Actively Care for Health and Safety

Second Edition

E. Scott Geller

LEWIS PUBLISHERS
Boca Raton London New York Washington, D.C.

Library of Congress Cataloging-in-Publication Data

Geller, E. Scott, 1942-
    Working safe : how to help people actively care for health and safety / E. Scott Geller.
        p. cm.
    Includes bibliographical references and index.
    Rev. and updated ed. of Working safe, c1996.
    Includes bibliographical references and index.
    ISBN 1-56670-564-9 (alk. paper)
    1. Industrial safety—Psychological aspects. I. Geller, E. Scott, 1942- Psychology of safety.
Selections. II. Title.

T55.3.B43 G452 2001
658.3′82′01—dc21
                                       2001020392
                                           CIP

Visit the CRC Press Web site at www.crcpress.com

© 2001 by CRC Press LLC
Lewis Publishers is an imprint of CRC Press LLC

No claim to original U.S. Government works
International Standard Book Number 1-56670-564-9
Library of Congress Card Number 2001020392
Printed in the United States of America   2 3 4 5 6 7 8 9 0
Printed on acid-free paper

Dedication

Past

to my mom (Margaret J. Scott) and dad (Edward I. Geller) who taught me the value of learning and reinforced my need to achieve.

to B. F Skinner and W. Edwards Deming who developed and researched the most applicable principles in this text, and inspired me to teach them.

Present

to my wife (Carol Ann) and mother-in-law (Betty Jane) whose continuous support for over 30 years made preparation to write this book possible.

to the students and associates in our university Center for Applied Behavior Systems whose data collection and analysis provided practical examples for the principles.

Future

to my daughters (Krista and Karly) who, I hope, will someday experience the sense of accomplishment I feel by completing this book.

to my seven associates at Safety Performance Solutions who, I hope, will continue to help corporations worldwide achieve a Total Safety Culture.

Preface

Working Safe teaches you about the psychology of safety in order to reduce the possibility of accidental injury to yourself and to others. Psychology influences every aspect of our lives, including our safety and health. And psychology can be used to benefit almost every aspect of our lives, including our safety and health.

So what is "psychology" anyway?

My *American Heritage Dictionary* (1991) defines psychology as "1. The science of mental processes and behavior and 2. The emotional and behavioral characteristics of an individual, group, or activity" (p. 1000). Similarly, the two definitions in the *New Merriam-Webster Dictionary* (1989) are "1. The science of mind and behavior and 2. The mental and behavioral characteristics of an individual or group" (p. 587).

In both dictionaries, the first definition of "psychology" uses the term "science" and refers to behavioral and mental processes. Behaviors are the outside, objective, and observable aspects of people; mental or mind reflects our inside, subjective, and unobservable characteristics. Science implies the application of the scientific method, or the objective and systematic analysis and interpretation of reliable observations of natural or experimental phenomena.

So what should you expect from a text on the psychology of safety? Obviously, such a book should show how psychology influences the safety and health of people. And to be useful, it should explain ways to apply psychology to improve safety and health. This is, in fact, my purpose for writing this text — to teach you how to use psychology both to explain and reduce personal injury.

As a science of mind and behavior, psychology is actually a vast field of numerous subdisciplines. Areas covered in a standard college course in introductory psychology, for example, include: research methods, physiological foundations, sensation and perception, language and thinking, consciousness and memory, learning, motivation and emotion, human development, intelligence, personality, psychological disorders, treatment of mental disorders, social thought and behavior, environmental psychology, and industrial/organizational psychology and human factors engineering. This book does not cover all of these areas of psychology, only those directly relevant to understanding and influencing safety-related behaviors and attitudes. In addition, my coverage of information within any one subdiscipline of psychology is not comprehensive, but focuses on only those aspects directly relevant to reducing injury in organizational and community settings.

This information will help you improve safety and health in any setting, from your home to the workplace and every community location in between. Actually, you can apply the knowledge gained from reading this book in all aspects of your daily life. Most organized safety-improvement efforts occur in work environments, however, because that's where the exposure to hazardous conditions and at-risk behavior is most obvious. As a result, most (but not all) of my illustrations and examples use an industrial context. My hope is that you will see direct relevance of the principles and procedures to domains beyond the workplace.

The human element of occupational health and safety is an extremely popular topic at national and regional safety conferences. Safety leaders realize that reducing injuries to below current levels requires increased attention to human factors. Engineering interventions and government policies have made their mark. Now it's time to include a focus on the human dynamics of injury prevention — *the psychology of safety*.

A comprehensive perspective

Most attempts to deal with the human aspects of safety have been limited in scope. Many trainers and consultants claim to have answers to the human side of safety, but their solutions are too often impractical, shortsighted, or illusory. And to support their particular program, consultants, authors, and conference speakers often give unfair and inaccurate criticism of alternative methods.

Tools from behavior-based safety have been criticized in an attempt to justify a focus on people's attitudes or values. In contrast, promoters of behavior-based safety have ridiculed a focus on attitudes as being too subjective, unscientific, and unrealistic. And both behavior-based and attitude-oriented approaches to injury prevention have been faulted in order to vindicate a systems- or culture-based approach. The truth of the matter is that both behaviors and attitudes require attention in order to develop large-scale and long-term improvement in people's safety and health.

There are a number of books on the market that offer advice regarding the human element of occupational safety. Unfortunately, many of these texts offer a limited perspective. And I've found none comprehensive and practical enough to show how to integrate behavior- and attitude-based perspectives for a system-wide total culture transformation. This book was written to do just that, and in this regard, it's one of a kind.

Simply put, behavioral science principles provide the basic tools and procedures for building an improved safety system. But the people in a work culture need to accept and use these behavior-based techniques appropriately. This is where a broader perspective is needed, including insight regarding more subjective concepts like attitude, value, and thought processes. Recall that psychology includes the scientific study of both mind and behavior. Therefore, a practical book on the psychology of safety needs to teach science-based and feasible approaches to change what people think (attitude) and do (behavior) in order to achieve a Total Safety Culture.

Cultivating a Total Safety Culture

I refer to a Total Safety Culture throughout this text as the ultimate vision of a safety-improvement mission. In a Total Safety Culture everyone feels responsible for safety and pursues it on a daily basis. At work, employees go beyond "the call of duty" to identify environmental hazards and at-risk behaviors. Then they intervene to correct them. And safe work practices are supported with proper recognition procedures. In a Total Safety Culture, safety is not a priority that gets shifted according to situational demands. Rather, safety is a value linked to all situational priorities.

Obviously, building a Total Safety Culture requires a long-term continuous improvement process. It involves cultivating constructive change in both the behaviors and attitudes of everyone in the culture. This book provides you with principles and procedures to make this happen. Applying what you read here might not result in a Total Safety Culture. But it's sure to make a beneficial difference in your own safety and health, and in the safety and health of others you choose to help.

I refer to helping others as "actively caring." This book shows you how to increase the quality and quantity of your own and others' actively caring behavior. Indeed, actively caring is the key to safety improvement. The more people actively caring for the safety and health of others, the less remote is the achievement of our ultimate vision — a Total Safety Culture.

Who should read this book?

My editor has warned me that one book can serve only a limited audience. I know he's right, but at the same time a practical book on reducing injuries is relevant for everyone. All of us risk personal injury of some sort during the course of our days, and all of us can do something to reduce that risk to ourselves and others. Therefore, a book that teaches practical ways to do this is pertinent reading for everyone.

The average person, however, won't spend valuable time reading a book on ways to reduce personal risk for injury. In fact, most people don't believe they are at risk for personal injury. So why should they read a book about improving safety? While I believe everyone *should* read this book, a text on the psychology of safety is destined for a select and elite audience: people who are concerned about the rate of injuries in their organizations or communities and want to do something about it.

This book is a second edition of a "best seller" book in occupational safety published in 1996. Every chapter has been updated and expanded, and three new chapters have been added — one on behavioral safety analysis, another on intervening with supportive conversation, and a third on promoting high-performance teamwork.

I am sensitive to the fact that new editions should justify their existence. I believe it's unfair to prepare another edition of a book that is not a significant improvement over an earlier edition, although I've seen this happen many times. I've often purchased a follow-up edition to a book only to find very little difference between the two versions. This is frequently the case with college textbooks.

This book offers more information than the 1996 version. Thus, readers of the first edition won't be disappointed if they purchase this revision. Plus, there are many potential applications of this text. It's a comprehensive source of psychological principles and practical applications for the safety professional or corporate safety leader. And it could be used as required or recommended reading in a number of undergraduate or graduate courses. More specifically, this book is ideal for courses on human factors engineering, safety management, or organizational performance management.

Many engineering and psychology departments do not offer courses with safety or human factors in their titles. However, this text is quite suitable for such standard courses as applied psychology, organizational psychology, management systems, engineering psychology, applied engineering, and even introductory psychology.

Fun to read

The writing style and format of this book are different from any professional text I have written or read. Most authors of professional books, including me, have been taught a particular academic or research style of writing that is not particularly enjoyable to read. When did you last pick up a nonfiction technical book for recreational or "fun" reading?

To attract more readership, this text is written in a more exciting style than most professional books, thanks to invaluable editorial coaching by Dave Johnson, editor of *Industrial Safety and Hygiene News*. Each chapter includes several original drawings by George Wills to illustrate concepts and add some humor to the learning process. I intersperse these drawings in my professional addresses and workshops, and audiences find them both enjoyable and enlightening.

I predict some of you will page through the book and look for these illustrations. That's a useful beginning to learning concepts and techniques for improving the human dynamics of safety. Then read the explanatory text for a second useful step toward making a difference with this information. If you then discuss the principles and procedures with others, you'll be on your way to putting this information to work in your organization, community, or home.

A testimony

Throughout this book, I include personal anecdotes to supplement the rationale of a principle or the description of a technique or process. I'd like to end this preface with one such anecdote. In August 1994, the Hercules Portland Plant stopped chemical production for two consecutive days so all 64 employees at the facility could attend a two-day workshop on the psychology of safety.

Management had received a request for this all-employee workshop from a team of hourly workers who previously attended my two-day professional development conference sponsored by the Mt. St. Helena Section of the American Society of Safety Engineers. Rick Moreno, a Hercules warehouse operator and hazardous materials unloader for more than 20 years, wrote the following reaction to my workshop. He read it to his coworkers at the start of the Hercules workshop. It set the stage for a most constructive and gratifying two days of education and training. If you approach the information in this book with some of the enthusiasm and optimism reflected in Rick's words, you can't help but make a difference in someone's safety and health.

> *Knowledge is precious. It's like trying to carry water in your cupped hands to a thirsty friend. Ideas that were crystal clear upon hearing them tend to slip from your memory like water through the creases of your hands, and while you may have brought back enough water to wet your friend's lips, he will not enjoy the full drink that you were able to take.*

And so it is with this analogy of the Total Safety Culture. Those who were there can only wet your lips with this new concept. Not a class or a program, but a safe, well way to live your life that spills into other avenues of our environment.

It has no limit or boundaries as in this year, this plant. It's more like we're on our way and something wonderful is going to happen.

And even though no answers are promised or given, the avenues in which to find our own answers for our own problems will be within our reach. . . That is why it is important that everyone has the opportunity to take a full drink of the Total Safety Culture instead of having our lips wet. Something wonderful is going to happen.

This book is for you — Rick Moreno — and the many others who want to understand the psychology of safety and reduce personal injuries. I hope this material will be used as a source of principles and procedures you can return to for guidance and benchmarks along your innovative journey toward building a safer culture of more actively caring people.

E. Scott Geller
May, 2001

Acknowledgments

In December 1992, I purchased an attractive print of a newborn colt from an artist at Galeria San Juan, Puerto Rico. While the artist — Jan D'Esopo — was signing my print, I asked her how long it took to complete the original. "Twenty-five minutes or 25 years," she replied, "depending on how you look at it." "What do you mean?" I asked. "Well, it took me only 25 minutes to fill the canvas, but it took me 25 years of training and experience to prepare for the artistry."

I feel similarly about completing this book, which is a revision and expansion of the first edition published in 1996. While writing the first edition and this revision took substantial time, the effort pales in comparison to the many years of preparation supported by invaluable contributions from teachers, researchers, consultants, safety professionals, university colleagues, and countless university students.

Actually, I've been preparing to write this text since entering the College of Wooster in Wooster, Ohio in 1960. Almost all exams at this small liberal arts college required written discussion (rather than selecting an answer from a list of alternatives). Therefore, I received early experience and feedback in integrating concepts and research findings from a variety of sources. I was introduced to the scientific method at Wooster, and applied it to my own behavioral science research during both my junior and senior years.

Throughout five years of graduate education at Southern Illinois University in Carbondale, Illinois, I developed sincere respect and appreciation for the scientific method as the key to gaining profound knowledge. My primary areas of graduate study were learning, personality, social dynamics, and human information processing and decision making. The chairman of both my thesis and dissertation committees (Dr. Gordon F. Pitz) gave me special coaching in research methodology and data analysis, and refined my skills for professional writing.

In 1968, I was introduced to the principles and procedures of applied behavior analysis (the foundation of behavior-based safety) from one graduate course and a few visits to Anna State Hospital in Anna, Illinois, where two eminent scholars, Drs. Ted Ayllon and Nate Azrin, were conducting seminal research in this field. Those learning experiences (brief in comparison with all my other education) convinced me that behavior-focused psychology could make large-scale improvements in people's lives. This insight was to have dramatic influence on my future teaching, research, and scholarship.

I started my professional career in 1969 as Assistant Professor of Psychology at Virginia Polytechnic Institute and State University (Virginia Tech). With assistance from undergraduate and graduate students, I developed a productive laboratory and research program in cognitive psychology. My tenure and promotion to Associate

Professor was based entirely upon my professional scholarship in this domain. However, in the mid-1970s I became concerned that this laboratory work had limited potential for helping people. This conflicted with my personal mission to make beneficial large-scale differences in people's quality of life. Therefore I turned to another line of research.

Given my conviction that behavior-based psychology has the greatest potential for solving organizational and community problems, I focused my research on finding ways to make this happen. Inspired by the first Earth Day in April 1970, my students and I developed, evaluated, and refined a number of community-based techniques for increasing environment-constructive behaviors and decreasing environment-destructive behaviors. This prolific research program culminated with the 1982 Pergamon Press publication of *Preserving the Environment: New Strategies for Behavior Change*, which I co-authored with Drs. Richard A. Winett and Peter B. Everett.

Besides targeting environmental protection, my students and I applied behavior-based psychology to a number of other problem areas, including prison administration, school discipline, community theft, transportation management, and alcohol-impaired driving. In the mid-1970s we began researching strategies for increasing the use of vehicle safety belts. This led to a focus on the application of behavior-based psychology to prevent unintentional injury in organizational and community settings.

Perhaps this brief history of my professional education and experience legitimizes my authorship of a book on the psychology of safety. However, my purpose for providing this information is not so much to provide credibility but to acknowledge the vast number of individuals — teachers, researchers, colleagues, and students — who prepared me to write this book. Critical for this preparation were our numerous research projects (since 1970), which could not have been possible without dedicated contributions from hundreds of university students. My graduate students managed most of these field studies, and I'm truly grateful for their valuable talents and loyal efforts.

Financial support from a number of corporations and government agencies made our 30 years of intervention research possible. Over the years, we received significant research funds from the Alcohol, Drug Abuse, and Mental Health Administration, the Alcoholic Beverage Medical Research Foundation, Anheuser-Busch Companies, Inc., the Centers for Disease Control and Prevention, Domino's Pizza, Inc., Exxon Chemical Company, General Motors Research Laboratories, Hoechst-Celanese, the Motor Vehicle Manufacturers Association, the Motors Insurance Corporation, the National Highway Traffic Safety Administration, the National Institute on Alcohol Abuse and Alcoholism, the National Institute for Occupational Safety and Health, the National Science Foundation, Sara Lee Knit Products, the U.S. Department of Education, the U.S. Department of Energy, the U.S. Department of Health, Education, and Welfare, the U.S. Department of Transportation, and the Virginia Departments of Agriculture and Commerce, Litter Control, Motor Vehicles, and Welfare and Institutions. Profound knowledge is only possible through programmatic research, and these organizations made it possible for my students and me to develop and systematically evaluate ways to improve attitudes and behaviors throughout organizations and communities.

I am also indebted to the numerous guiding and motivating communications I have received from corporate and community safety professionals worldwide. Daily contacts with these individuals shaped my research and scholarship, and challenged me to improve the connection between research and application. They also provided valuable positive reinforcement to prevent "burnout." It would take pages to name all of these friends and acquaintances, and then I would necessarily miss many. You know who you are — thank you!

The advice, feedback, and friendship of two individuals — Harry Glaser and Dave Johnson — have been invaluable for my preparation to write this text. I first met Harry Glaser in September 1992 after I gave a keynote address at a professional development conference for the American Society of Safety Engineers. As Executive Vice President of Tel-A-Train, Inc., Harry decided that a video-training series on the human dynamics I presented in my talk would be useful. That was the start of ongoing collaboration in developing videotape scripts, training manuals, and facilitator guides — invaluable preparation for writing this text. In particular, my relationship with Harry Glaser improved my ability to communicate the practical implications of academic research and scholarship.

Also vital to bridging the gap between research and application has been my long-term alliance and synergism with Dave Johnson, Editor of *Industrial Safety and Hygiene News*. Dave and I began learning from each other in the Spring of 1990 when I submitted my first article for his magazine. That year I submitted five articles on the psychology of safety, and Dave did substantial editing on each. Every time one of my articles was published, I learned something about communicating the bottom line of a psychological principle or procedure more effectively.

As an author of more than 250 research articles and former Editor of the premier research journal in the applied behavioral sciences (*Journal of Applied Behavior Analysis*), I knew quite well how to write for a research audience in psychology. But Dave Johnson showed me that when it comes to writing for safety professionals and the general public, I had a lot to learn. And in this regard, I continue to learn from him. Beginning in 1994, I've written a monthly article for a "Psychology of Safety" column in *Industrial Safety and Hygiene News*. Each of these contributions profited immensely from Dave's suggestions and feedback. In fact, preparing those articles laid the groundwork for this book. Dave served as editor of the first edition of this text, dedicating long hours to improving the clarity and readability of my writing. Thus, the talent and insight of Dave Johnson have been incorporated throughout this text, and I am eternally beholden to him.

The illustrations throughout this book were drawn by George Wills of Blacksburg, VA, and I think they add vitality and fun to the written presentation. I hope you agree. But without the craft and dedication of Brian Lea, the illustrations could not have been combined with the text for use by the publisher. In fact, Brian coordinated the final processing of this entire text, combining tables and diagrams (which he refined) with George Wills' illustrations, and the word processing from Gayle Kennedy, Nick Buscemi, and Cassie Wright.

I also sincerely appreciate the daily support and encouragement I received from my graduate students in 2000: Chris Dula, Kelli England, Jeff Hickman, Rebecca Click Keeney, and Angie Krom; my colleagues at Safety Performance Solutions: Susan Bixler, Anne French, Mike Gilmore, Molly McClintock, Sherry Perdue, Chuck Pettinger, Steve Roberts, and Josh Williams; and from Kent Glindemann — Research Scientist for the Center for Applied Behavior Systems. Finally, I am indebted to the entire staff at CRC Press who brought this book to life, from acquisitions to editing, printing, distributing and marketing. Three individuals helped me most directly. Randi Gonzalez and Judith Kamin actively cared for the numerous details involved in getting my manuscript ready for publication. Arline Massey had the dynamic vision and thoughtful action plan to put the whole project in motion.

A terrible disease prevented Arline Massey from managing the process she started, and it took her life on New Year's Eve 2000. Words cannot reflect the sense of sadness and loss felt by her family, friends, and colleagues. I wanted so very much to thank Arline personally for making the book happen.

All of these people, plus many, many more, have contributed to 40 years of preparation for *Working Safe*. I thank you all very much. I hope the synergy from all your contributions will help readers make rewarding and long-term differences in people's lives.

E. Scott Geller
May, 2001

Author

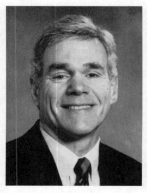 E. Scott Geller, Ph. D., is a Senior Partner with Safety Performance Solutions, Inc. — a leading-edge organization specializing in behavior-based safety training and consulting. Dr. Geller and his partners at Safety Performance Solutions (SPS) have helped companies across the country and around the world address the human dynamics of occupational safety through flexible research-founded principles and industry-proven tools. In addition, for more than three decades, Professor Geller has taught and conducted research as a faculty member in the Department of Psychology at Virginia Polytechnic Institute and State University, better known as Virginia Tech. In this capacity, he has authored more than 300 research articles and over 50 books or chapters addressing the development and evaluation of behavior-change interventions to improve quality of life.

His recent books in occupational health and safety include: *The Psychology of Safety Handbook*; *Understanding Behavior-Based Safety*; *Building Successful Safety Teams*; *Beyond Safety Accountability: How to Increase Personal Responsibility*; *The Psychology of Safety Handbook*; and the primer: *What Can Behavior-Based Safety Do for Me?*

Dr. Geller is a Fellow of the American Psychological Association, the American Psychological Society, and the World Academy of Productivity and Quality Sciences. He is past editor of the *Journal of Applied Behavior Analysis* (1989-1992), current associate editor of *Environment and Behavior* (since 1983), and current consulting editor for *Behavior and Social Issues*, the *Behavior Analyst Digest*, the *Journal of Organizational Behavior Management*, and the *International Journal of Behavioral Safety*.

Geller earned a teaching award in 1982 from the American Psychological Association, as well as every university teaching award offered at Virginia Tech. In 1983 he received the Virginia Tech Alumni Teaching Award and was elected to the Virginia Tech Academy of Teaching Excellence; in 1990 he was honored with the university Sporn Award for distinguished teaching of freshman level courses, and in 1999 he was awarded the prestigious W. E. Wine Award for Teaching Excellence.

Dr. Geller has written over 100 articles for *Industrial Safety and Hygiene News*, a trade magazine disseminated to more than 75,000 companies. Dr. Geller has been the principal investigator for more than 75 research grants that have involved the application of behavioral science for the benefit of corporations, institutions, government agencies, and communities.

Contents

part one

Orientation and alignment

chapter one

Choosing the right approach

The basic purpose of this book is outlined in this chapter: to explore the human dynamics of occupational health and safety, and to show how they can be managed to significantly improve safety performance. The principles and practical procedures you will learn are based on neither common sense nor intuition, but rather on reliable scientific investigation. Many recommendations seem counter to "pop psychology" and traditional approaches to safety. So keep an open mind while you read about the psychology of safety.

"Organizations learn only through individuals who learn." — Peter Senge

Safety professionals, team leaders, and concerned workers today scramble to find the "best" safety approach for their workplace. Typically, whatever offers the cheapest "quick fix" sells. This is not surprising, given the "lean and mean" atmosphere of the times. Programs that offer the most benefit with least effort sound best, but will they really work to improve safety over the long term?

This text will help you ask the right questions to determine whether a particular approach to safety improvement will work. More importantly, this text describes the basic ingredients needed to improve organizational and community safety. In fact, you will find sufficient information to improve any safety process. Learning the principles and procedures described here will enable you to make a beneficial, long-term difference in the safety and health of your workplace, home, and community. The information is relevant for most other performance domains, from increasing the quantity and quality of productivity in the workplace to improving quality of life in homes, neighborhoods, and throughout entire communities.

Selecting the best approach

With so many different approaches to safety improvement available, how can we select the best? My first thought is to ask, "What does the research indicate?" In other words, are there objective data available from program comparisons to shed light on our dilemma? Unfortunately, there are few systematic comparisons of alternative safety interventions. However, this does not stop consultants from showing us impressive results regarding the success of their approaches. Nor does it prevent them from

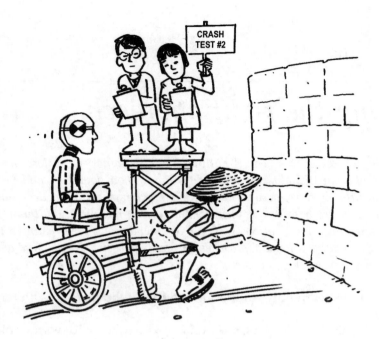

Figure 1.1 Some research is not worth considering.

implying (or boldly stating) that we can obtain similar fantastic results by simply following their patented "steps to success."

Keep in mind this marketing information usually comes from selected client case studies. Very few of these "success stories" were collected objectively and reliably enough to meet the rigorous standards of a professional research journal. When consultants try to sell you an approach to safety with this kind of data, ask them if they have published their results in a peer-reviewed journal. If they can show you a published research report of their impressive results or a professional presentation of a program very similar to theirs, then give their approach special consideration in your selection process. The validity and applicability of even published research varies dramatically, however. Figure 1.1 depicts the low end of research quality.

Most of the published research on safety improvement systematically evaluates whether a particular program worked in a particular situation, but it does not compare one approach with another. In other words, this research tells us whether a certain strategy is better than nothing, but offers no information regarding the relative impact of two or more different strategies on safety improvement. Such research has limited usefulness when selecting among different approaches.

An exception can be found in a review article in *Safety Science*, where Stephen Guastello (1993) summarized systematically the evaluation data from 53 different research reports of safety programs. Guastello provided rare and useful information for deciding how to improve safety. You can assume the evaluations were both reliable and valid, because each report appeared in a scientific peer-reviewed journal. All of the studies selected for his summary were conducted in a workplace setting since 1977, and each study evaluated program impact with outcome data (including number and severity of injuries).

From my reading of Guastello's article, I believe it is safe to say the behavior-based and comprehensive ergonomics approaches lead the field. Personnel selection, the most popular method (26 studies targeted a total of 19,177 employees), is among the least effective. Here are brief descriptions of these approaches to reduce workplace injuries, ranked according to their effectiveness.

Behavior-based programs

Programs in this category consisted of employee training regarding particular safe and at-risk behaviors, systematic observation and recording of the targeted behaviors, and feedback to workers regarding the frequency or percentage of safe vs. at-risk behavior. Some of these programs included goal setting and/or incentives to encourage the observation and feedback process.

Comprehensive ergonomics

The ergonomics (or human factors) approach to safety refers essentially to any adjustment of working conditions or equipment in order to reduce the frequency or probability of an environmental hazard or at-risk behavior. An essential ingredient in these programs was a diagnostic survey or environmental audit by employees which led to specific recommendations for eliminating hazards that put employees at risk or promoted at-risk behaviors.

Engineering changes

This category includes the introduction of robots or the comprehensive redesign of facilities to eliminate certain at-risk behaviors. It is noted, however, that the robotic interventions introduced the potential for new types of workplace injuries, like a robot catching an operator in its work envelope and impaling him or her against a structure. Thus, robotic innovations usually require additional engineering intervention such as equipment guards, emergency kill switches, radar-type sensors, and workplace redesign to prevent injury from robots. Behavioral training, observation, and feedback (as detailed in Part 4 of this book) are also needed following engineering redesign.

Group problem solving

For this approach, operations personnel met voluntarily to discuss safety issues and problems, and to develop action plans for safety improvement. This approach is analogous to quality circles where employees who perform similar types of work meet regularly to solve problems of product quality, productivity, and cost.

Government action (in Finland)

In Finland, two government agencies responsible for labor production target the most problematic occupational groups and implement certain action strategies.

These include:

1. Disseminating information to work supervisors regarding the causes of work-place injuries and methods to reduce them
2. Setting standards for safe machine repair and use and
3. Conducting periodic work site inspections

Management audits

For the programs in this category, designated managers were trained to administer a standard International Safety Rating System (ISRS). This system evaluates workplaces based on 20 components of industrial safety. These include leadership and administration, management training, planned inspections, task and procedures analysis, task observations, emergency preparedness, organizational rules, accident analysis, employee training, personal protective equipment, health control, program evaluation, engineering controls, and off-the-job safety.

Managers conduct the comprehensive audits annually to develop improvement strategies for the next year. Specially certified ISRS personnel visit target sites and recognize a plant with up to five "stars" for exemplary safety performance.

Stress management

These programs taught employees how to cope with stressors or sources of work stress. Exercise was often a key action strategy promoted as a way to prevent stress-related injuries in physically demanding jobs. I discuss the topic of stress as it relates to injury prevention in Chapter 6.

Poster campaigns

The two published studies in this category evaluated the accident reduction impact of posting signs that urged workers at a shipyard to avoid certain at-risk behaviors and to follow certain safe behaviors. Most signs were posted at relevant locations and gave specific behavioral instructions like "Take material for only one workday," "Gather hoses immediately after use," "Wear your safety helmet," and "Check railing and platform couplings (on scaffolds)."

For one study, safety personnel at the shipyard gave work teams weekly feedback regarding compliance with sign instructions. In the other study, environmental audits, group discussions, and structured interviews were used to develop the poster messages. Thus, it's possible that factors other than the posters themselves contributed to the moderate short-term impact of this intervention approach. All of these factors are covered in this book, including ways to maximize the beneficial effects of safety signs (in Chapter 10).

Personnel selection

This popular but ineffective approach to injury prevention is based on the intuitive notion of "accident proneness." The strategy is to identify aspects of accident proneness among job applicants and then screen out people with critical levels of certain characteristics.

Although measuring and screening for accident proneness sounds like a "quick fix" approach to injury prevention, this method has several problems you will readily realize as you read more in this book about the psychology of safety. Briefly, this technique has not worked reliably to prevent workplace injuries because:

1. The instruments or procedures available to measure the proneness character-istics are unreliable or invalid.
2. The characteristics do not carry across settings, so a person might show them at home but not at work or vice versa.
3. A person with a higher desire to take risks (such as a sensation seeker) might be less inclined to take appropriate precautions (like using personal protective equipment) to avoid potential injury.

"Near-miss" reporting

This approach involved increased reporting and investigation of incidents that did not result in an injury but certainly could have under slightly different circumstances. One program in this category increased the number of corrective suggestions gener-ated but did not reduce injury rate. The other scientific publication in this category reported a 56 percent reduction in injury *severity* as a result of increased reporting of near hits,* but the overall *number* of injuries did not change.

The critical human element

Every safety approach described above requires that you consider the human element or the psychology of safety. Indeed, the most successful approaches, behavior-based safety and comprehensive ergonomics, directly address the human aspects of safety. The bottom line is illustrated in Figure 1.2. The three employees here are looking at a contributing factor in almost every injury — the human factor. Thus, any safety intervention that improves the safety-related behaviors of workers will prevent workplace injuries.

The behavior-based approach targets human behavior and relies on interpersonal observation and feedback for intervention. The success of comprehensive ergonomics depends on employees observing relationships between behaviors and work situa-tions, and then recommending feasible changes in behavior, equipment, or environ-mental conditions to make the job more "user friendly" and safe.

Today, achieving success in safety requires concerted efforts in the realm of psy-chology. Safety professionals are hungry for insights. In recent years, many seminars at national and regional safety conferences purporting to teach aspects of the psychology of safety attracted standing-room only crowds. Just look at these titles from recent conferences of the National Safety Council or the American Society of Safety Engineers.

*   Managing Safe Behavior for Lasting Change
*   Humanizing the Total Safety Program
*   The Human Element in Achieving a Total Safety Culture

---

* "Near miss" is used routinely in the workplace to refer to an incident that did not result in an injury. Since a literal translation of this term means the injury actually occurred, "near hit" is used throughout this book instead of "near miss."

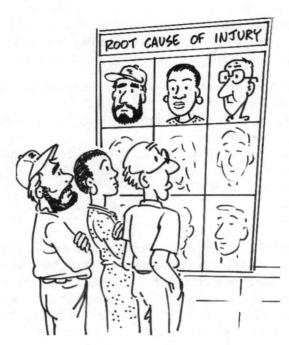

Figure 1.2 Human dynamics contribute to almost every injury.

- The Psychology of Injury Prevention
- Behavior-Based Safety Management: Parallels with the Quality Process
- Behavioral Management Techniques for Continuous Improvement
- Improving Safety through Innovative Behavioral and Cultural Approaches
- Safety Leadership Power: How to Empower All Employees
- Moving to the Second Generation in Behavior-Based Safety
- Potholes in the Road to Behavioral Safety
- Implementing Behavior-Based Safety on a Large Scale
- Motivating Employees for Safety Success
- Integrating Behavioral Safety into Other Safety Management Systems
- From Knowing to Doing: Achieving Safety Excellence
- Safety and Psychology: Where Do We Go from Here?

I attended each of these presentations and found numerous inconsistencies between presentations dealing with the same topic. Sometimes, I noted erroneous and frivolous statements, inaccurate or incomplete reference to psychological theory or research, and invalid or irresponsible comparisons between various approaches to dealing with the psychology of safety. It seemed a primary aim of several presentations was to "sell" their own particular programs or consulting services by overstating the benefits of their approach and giving an incomplete or naive discussion of alternative methods or procedures.

The folly of choosing what sounds good

The theory, research, and tools in psychology are so vast and often so complex that it can be overwhelming to decide which particular approach or strategy to use. As a

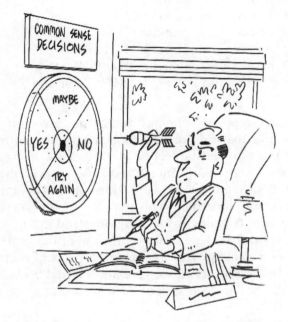

Figure 1.3 Without science, decision making is a biased shot in the dark.

result, we are easily biased by common-sense words that sound good. As depicted in Figure 1.3, common sense is subjective, based on a person's everyday *selective* experiences and biased interpretations of those experiences.

Valid theory, principles, and procedures founded on solid research evidence are often ignored. Today, there seems to be an apparently endless market of self-help books, audiotapes, and videotapes addressing concepts seemingly relevant to the psychology of injury prevention. In recent years, I have listened to the following audiotapes — representing only a fraction of "pop psychology" tapes with topics relevant to the psychology of safety:

- "Coping with Difficult People" by R. M. Branson
- "Personal Excellence" by K. Blanchard
- "How to Build High Self-Esteem" by J. Canfield
- "The Seven Habits of Highly Effective People" by S. R. Covey
- "First Things First" by S. R. Covey, A. R. Merrill, and R. R. Merrill
- "The Science of Personal Achievement" by N. Hill
- "Increasing Human Effectiveness" by R. Moawad
- "Lead the Field" by E. Nightingale
- "Unlimited Power" by A. Robbins
- "The Psychology of Achievement" by B. Tracey
- "The Psychology of Success" by B. Tracey
- "The Universal Laws of Success and Achievement" by B. Tracy
- "The Psychology of Winning" by D. Waitley
- "Self-Esteem" by J. White
- "Goal Setting" by Z. Ziglar

- "Top Performance" by Z. Ziglar
- "The Secrets of Power Persuasion" by R. Dawson
- "The 12 Life Secrets" by R. Stuberg
- "The Courage to Live Your Dreams" by L. Brown
- "The New Dynamics of Goal Setting" by D. Waitley
- "Transforming Stress into Power" by M. J. Tazer and S. Willard

Which, if any, of these pop psychology audiotapes gives safety professionals the "truth" — the most effective and practical tools for dealing with the human aspects of safety? Some of the most cost-effective strategies for managing behaviors and attitudes at the personal and organizational level are not even mentioned in many of the pop psychology books, audiotapes, and videotapes. This might be the case not only because authors and presenters are unaware of the latest research, but also because many of the best techniques for individual and group improvement do not sound good — at least at first. The primary purpose of this text is to teach the most effective approaches for dealing with the human aspects of occupational safety and health. These principles and procedures were not selected because they sound good, but because their validity has been supported with sound research.

Relying on research

This book teaches research-based psychology related to occupational safety. Thus, by reading this text you'll improve your common sense about the psychology of safety. At this point, I hope you are open to questioning the validity of good-sounding statements that are not supported by sound research.

Research in psychology, for example, does not generally support the following common statements related to the psychology of occupational health and safety:

- Practice makes perfect.
- Spare the rod and spoil the child.
- Attitudes need to be changed before behavior will change.
- Human nature motivates safe and healthy behavior.
- People will naturally help in a crisis.
- Rewards for not having injuries reduce injuries.
- All injuries are preventable.
- Zero injuries should be a safety goal.
- Manage only that which can be measured.
- Safety should be considered a priority.

These and other common safety beliefs will be refuted in this book, with reference to scientific knowledge obtained from systematic research. Sometimes, case studies will illustrate the practicality and benefits of a particular principle or procedure, but the validity of the information was not founded on case studies alone. The approaches presented in this text were originally discovered and verified with systematic and repeated scientific research in laboratory and field settings.

Start with behavior

Many pop psychology self-help books, audiotapes, and motivational speeches give minimal if any attention to behavior-based approaches to personal achievement. "Behavioral control" and "behavior modification" do not sound good. The term "behavior" has negative connotations, as in "let's talk about your behavior at the party last night." Dr. B. F. Skinner, the founder of behavioral science and its many practical applications, was one of the most misunderstood and underappreciated scientists and scholars of this century, primarily because the behavior management principles he taught did not sound good.

Professor Skinner and his followers have shown over and over again that behavior is motivated by its consequences, and thus behavior can be changed by controlling the events that follow behavior (e.g., see Skinner, 1979). But this principle of "control by consequences" does not sound as good as "control by positive thinking and free will." Therefore, the scientific principles and procedures from behavioral science have been underappreciated and underused.

This book teaches you how to apply behavioral science for safety achievement. The research recommends we start with behavior. But the demonstrated validity of a behavior-based approach does not mean the better-sounding, person-based approaches should not be used. It's important to consider the feelings and attitudes of employees, because it takes people to implement the tools of behavior management.

This text will teach you how certain feeling states critical for safety achievement — self-esteem, empowerment, and belonging — can be increased by applying behavioral science. It's possible to establish interpersonal interactions and behavioral consequences in the workplace to increase important feelings and attitudes. I will show you how increasing these feeling states benefits behavior and helps to achieve safety excellence.

As illustrated in Figure 1.4, an attitude of frustration or an internal state of distress can certainly influence driving behaviors, and vice versa. Indeed, internal (unobserved) personal states of mind continually influence observable behaviors, while changes in observable behaviors continually affect changes in person states or attitudes. Thus, it is possible to "think a person into safe behaviors" (through education, coaching, and consensus-building exercises), and it is possible to "act a person into safe thinking" (through behavior management techniques).

In an industrial setting, it is most cost effective to target behaviors first through behavior management interventions (described in this text) implemented by employees themselves. Small changes in behavior can result in attitude change, followed by more behavior change and more desired attitude change. This spiraling of behavior feeding attitude, attitude feeding behavior, behaviors feeding attitudes and so on can lead to employees becoming totally committed to safety achievement, as reflected in their daily behavior. And all of this could start with a relatively insignificant behavior change in one employee — a "small win."

In conclusion

In this initial chapter, I have outlined the basic purpose of this text, which is to teach principles for understanding the human aspects of occupational health and safety,

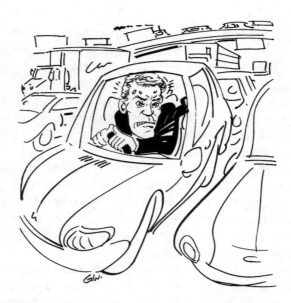

Figure 1.4 Behavior influences attitude and attitude influences behavior.

and to illustrate practical procedures for applying these principles to achieve significant improvements in organizational and community-wide safety.

The principles and procedures are not based on common sense or intuition, but
rather on reliable scientific investigation. Some will contradict common folklore in
pop psychology and require shifts in traditional approaches to the management of
organizational safety. Approach this material with an open mind. Be ready to relinquish fads, fancies, and folklore for innovations based on unpopular but research-
supported theory.

I promise this "psychology of safety" is based on the latest and most reliable
scientific knowledge related to individual and organizational safety. As illustrated in
Figure 1.5, "trying harder" cannot substitute for proper equipment, method, and tools.
This book provides research-tested methods and tools for improving the human
dynamics of safety, and thereby preventing injuries at work, at home, and throughout
your community.

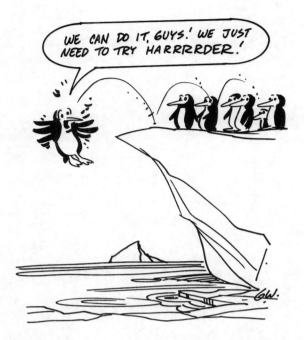

Figure 1.5 Motivation cannot substitute for equipment and method.

chapter two

Starting with theory

In this chapter we consider the value of theory in guiding our approaches to safety and health improvement. You will see how a vision for a Total Safety Culture is a necessary guide to achieve safety excellence. A basic principle here is that safety performance results from the dynamic interaction of environment, behavior, and person-based factors. Achieving a Total Safety Culture requires attention to each of these. I make a case for integrating person-based and behavior-based psychology in order to address most effectively the human dynamics of injury prevention.

"There's nothing so practical as a good theory." — Kurt Lewin

As you know, some safety efforts suffer from a "flavor of the month" syndrome. New procedures or intervention programs are tried seemingly at random, without an apparent vision, plan, or supporting set of principles. When the mission and principles are not clear, employees' acceptance and involvement suffer.

A theory or set of guiding principles makes it possible to evaluate the consistency and validity of program goals and intervention strategies. By summarizing the appropriate theory or principles into a mission statement, you have a standard for judging the value of your company's procedures, policies, and performance expectations.

It's important to develop a set of comprehensive principles on which to base safety procedures and policies. Then teach these principles to your employees so they are understood, accepted, and appreciated. This buy-in is certainly strengthened when employees or associates help select the safety principles to follow and summarize them in a company mission statement.

This is theory-based safety. A critical challenge, of course, is to choose the most relevant theories or principles for your company culture and purpose, and develop an appropriate and feasible mission statement that reflects the right theory.

The mission statement

Several years ago I worked with employees of a major chemical company to develop the general mission statement for safety given in Figure 2.1. This vision for a Total Safety Culture serves as a guideline or standard for the material presented throughout this book, in the same way a corporate mission statement serves as a yardstick for gauging the development and implementation of policies and procedures.

Mission Statement

A Total Safety Culture (TSC) continually improves safety performance. To that end, a TSC:

Promotes a work environment based on employee involvement, ownership, team work, education, training, and leadership.

Builds self–esteem, empowerment, pride, enthusiasm, optimism, and encourages innovation.

Reinforces the need for employees to actively care about their fellow coworkers.

Promotes the philosophy that safety is not a priority that can be reordered, but is a value associated with every priority.

Recognizes group and individual achievement.

Figure 2.1 The principles and procedures covered in this book are reflected in this safety achievement mission statement.

This mission statement might not be suited for all organizations, but it is based on appropriate and comprehensive theory, supported by scientific data from research in psychology. Before developing this statement, employees learned basic psychological theories most relevant to improving occupational safety. These principles are illustrated throughout this text, along with operational (real-world) definitions.

Theory as a map

I would like to relate an experience to show how a theory can be seen as a map to guide us to a destination. The mission statement in Figure 2.1 reflects a destination for safety within the realm of psychology. This story also reflects the difficulty in finding the best theory among numerous possibilities.

I had the opportunity to conduct a training program at a company in Palatka, FL. My client sent me step-by-step instructions to take me from Interstate 95 to Palatka. That was my map, limited in scope for sure, but sufficient I presumed to get the job done — to get me to the Holiday Inn in Palatka. But while at the National Car Rental desk, an attendant said my client's directions were incorrect and showed me the "correct way" with National's map of Jacksonville.

I was quick to give up my earlier theory (from my client's handwritten instructions) for this more professional display. After all, I now had a professionally printed map and directions from someone in the business of helping customers with travel plans — a consultant, so to speak. But National's map showed details for a limited

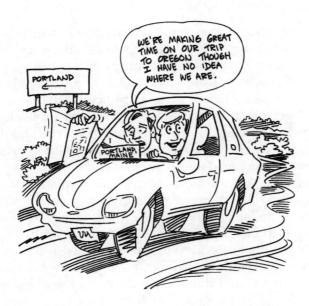

Figure 2.2 Start your journey with the right theory.

area, and Palatka was not on the map. I could not verify the attendant's directions with the map, nor could I compare these directions with my client's very different instructions. Without a complete perspective, I chose the theory that looked better. And I got lost. As depicted in Figure 2.2, it is critical to start out with the right map (or theory).

After traveling 15 miles, I began to question the "National theory" and wondered whether my client's scribbling had been correct after all. But I stuck by my decision, and drove another ten miles before exiting the highway in search of further instruction. I certainly needed to reach my destination that night, but motivation without appropriate direction can do more harm than good. In other words, a motivated worker cannot reach safety goals with the wrong theory or principles.

It was late Sunday night and the gas station off the exit ramp was closed, but another vehicle had also just stopped in the parking lot. I drove closer and announced to four tough-looking, grubby characters in a pick-up truck loaded with motorcycles that I was lost and wondered if they knew how to get to Palatka. None of these men had heard of Palatka, but one pulled out a detailed map of Florida and eventually found the town of Palatka. I could not see the details in the dark, but I accepted this new "theory" anyway, with no personal verification.

The packaging of this theory was not impressive, but my back was against the wall. I was desperate for a solution to my problem and had no other place to turn. As I left the parking lot with a new theory, I wondered whether I was now on the right track. Perhaps, the theory obtained from the National Car rental attendants was correct and I had missed an exit. Whom should I believe? Fortunately, I looked beyond the slick packaging and went with the guy who had the more comprehensive perspective (the larger map). This theory got me to the Holiday Inn Palatka.

Relevance to occupational safety

That evening I thought about my experience and its relevance to safety. It reminded me of the dilemma facing many safety professionals when they choose approaches, programs, and consultants to help solve people problems related to safety. Theories, research, and tools in psychology are so vast and often so complex that it can be an overwhelming task to select a theory or set of principles to follow.

The theory that got me to Palatka was not the most professional or believable, nor was it "packaged" impressively. This does not mean you should avoid the slick, well-marketed approaches to occupational safety. I only wish these factors were given much less weight than scientific data.

It is relevant, though, that the more comprehensive map enabled me to find my destination. I have found that many of the human approaches to improving safety are limited in scope or theoretical foundation. Many are sold or taught as packaged programs or step-by-step procedures for any workplace culture.

In the long run, it's more useful to teach comprehensive theory and principles. On this foundation, culture-relevant procedures and interventions can be crafted by employees who will "own" and thus follow them. As the old saying goes, "Give a man a fish and you feed him for a day; teach him how to fish and you feed him for a lifetime."

At breakfast, I told the human resource manager and the safety director, the one who gave me the handwritten instructions, about my problems finding Palatka. Interestingly, each had a different theory on the best way to travel between the Jacksonville airport and Palatka. The safety director stuck with his initial instructions. The human resource manager recommended the route I eventually took. Their discussion was not enlightening. In fact it got me more confused, because I did not have a visual picture or schema (a comprehensive map) in which to fit the various approaches (or routes) they were discussing. In other words, I did not have a framework or paradigm to organize their verbal descriptions. Without a relevant theory my experience taught me nothing, except the need for an appropriate theory — in this case a map.

A theory should serve as the map that provides direction to meet a specific safety challenge. Obviously, it's important to teach the basic theory to everyone who must meet the challenge. Then it is a good idea to have an employee task force summarize the theory in a safety mission statement. When the work force understands the theory and accepts the summary mission statement, intervention processes based on the theory will not be viewed as "flavor of the month," but as an action plan to bring the theory to life.

When employees appreciate and affirm the theory, they will get involved in designing and implementing the action steps. They will also suggest ways to refine or expand action plans and theory on the basis of systematic observations or scientific evidence. This is the best kind of continuous improvement.

A basic mission and theory

The mission statement in Figure 2.1 reflects the ultimate in safety — a Total Safety Culture. In a Total Safety Culture:

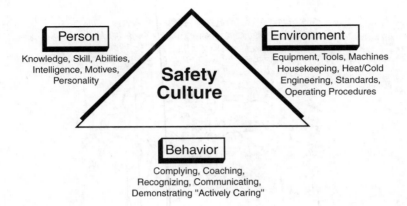

Figure 2.3 A Total Safety Culture requires constant attention
to three types of continuing factors.

- Everyone feels responsible for safety and does something about it on a daily basis.
- People go beyond the call of duty to identify unsafe conditions and at-risk behaviors, and they intervene to correct them.
- Safe work practices are supported intermittently with rewarding feedback from both peers and managers.
- People "actively care" continuously for the safety of themselves and others.
- Safety is not considered a priority that can be conveniently shifted depending on the demands of the situation; rather, safety is considered a value linked with every priority of a given situation.

This Total Safety Culture mission is much easier said than done, but it is achievable through a variety of safety processes rooted in the disciplines of engineering and psychology. Generally, a Total Safety Culture requires continual attention to three domains:

1. Environment factors (including equipment, tools, physical layout, procedures, standards, and temperature)
2. Person factors (including people's attitudes, beliefs, and personalities)
3. Behavior factors (including safe and at-risk work practices, as well as going beyond the call of duty to intervene on behalf of another person's safety)

This triangle of safety-related factors is illustrated in Figure 2.3. The various factors are dynamic and interactive. Changes in one domain eventually impact the other two. For example, behaviors that reduce the probability of injury often involve environmental change and lead to attitudes consistent with the safe behaviors. The behavior and person factors represent the human dynamics of occupational safety and are addressed in this book.

Paying attention to only behavior-based factors (the observable activities of people) or to only person-based factors (unobservable feeling states or attitudes of people) is like using a limited map to find a destination, as with my attempt to find Palatka,

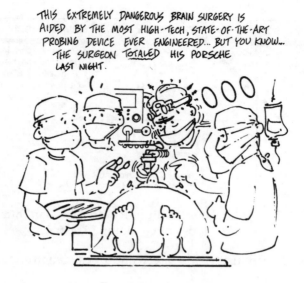

Figure 2.4 Performance results from the dynamic interaction of environment, behavior, and person factors.

FL. The mission to achieve a Total Safety Culture requires a comprehensive framework — a complete map of the relevant psychological territory. Figure 2.4 illustrates the complex interaction of environment, person, and behavior factors.

Behavior-based vs. person-based approaches

There are numerous opinions and recommendations on how the psychology of safety can be used to produce beneficial changes in people and organizations. Most can be classified into one of two basic approaches: person-based and behavior-based. In fact, most of the numerous psychotherapies available to treat developmental disabilities and psychological disorders, from neurosis to psychosis, can be classified as essentially person-based or behavior-based.

That is, most psychotherapies focus on changing people either from the inside ("thinking people into acting differently") or from the outside ("acting people into thinking differently"). Person-based approaches attack individual attitudes or thinking processes directly. They teach clients new thinking strategies or give them insight into the origin of their abnormal or unhealthy thoughts, attitudes, or feelings. In contrast, behavior-based approaches attack a client's behaviors directly. They change relationships between behaviors and their consequences. This text will show you how to integrate relevant principles from these two psychological approaches in order to achieve a Total Safety Culture.

The person-based approach

Imagine you see two employees pushing each other in a parking lot as a crowd gathers around to watch. Is this aggressive behavior, horseplay, or mutual instruction for self-defense? Are the employees physically attacking each other to inflict harm or does this physical contact indicate a special friendship and mutual understanding of the line between aggression and play? Perhaps if you watch longer and pay attention to verbal behavior, you will decide whether this is aggression, horseplay, or a teaching/ learning demonstration.

However, a truly accurate account might require you to assess each individual's personal feelings, attitudes, or intentions. It's possible, in fact, that one person was being hostile while the other was just having fun, or the contact started as horseplay and progressed to aggression.

This scenario illustrates a basic premise of the person-based approach. Focusing only on observable behavior does not explain enough. People are much more than their behaviors. Concepts like intention, creativity, intrinsic motivation, subjective interpretation, self-esteem, and mental attitude are essential to understanding and appreciating the human dynamics of a problem. Thus, a person-based approach in the workplace applies surveys, personal interviews, and focus-group discussions to find out how individuals feel about certain situations, conditions, behaviors, or personal interactions.

Humanism is the most popular person-based approach today, as evidenced by the current market of pop psychology videotapes, audiotapes, and self-help books. The key principles of humanism found in most pop psychology approaches to increase personal achievement are:

1. Everyone is unique in numerous ways. The special characteristics of individuals cannot be understood or appreciated by applying general principles or concepts, such as the behavior-based principles of performance management or the permanent personality trait perspective of psychoanalysis.
2. Individuals have far more potential to achieve than they typically realize and should not feel hampered by past experiences or present liabilities.
3. The present state of an individual in terms of feeling, thinking, and believing is a critical determinant of personal success.
4. One's self-concept influences mental and physical health, as well as personal effectiveness and achievement.
5. Ineffectiveness and abnormal thinking and behavior result from large discrepancies between one's real self ("who I am") and ideal self ("who I would like to be").
6. Individual motives vary widely and come from within a person.

The behavior-based approach

The behavior-based approach to applied psychology is founded on behavioral science as conceptualized and researched by B. F. Skinner (1938, 1974). In his experimental analysis of behavior, Professor Skinner rejected *for scientific study* unobservable factors such as self-esteem, intentions, and attitudes. He researched only observable behavior and its social, environmental, and physiological determinants. The behavior-based approach starts by identifying observable behaviors targeted for change and the environmental conditions that can be manipulated to influence the target behavior(s) in desired directions.

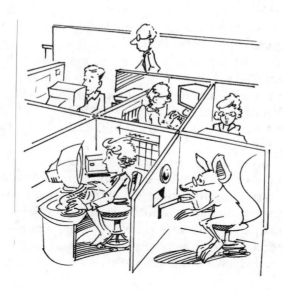

Figure 2.5 It is an S-R world after all.

The basic idea is that behavior can be objectively studied and changed by iden-tifying and manipulating environmental conditions (or stimuli) that immediately precede and follow a target behavior. The antecedent conditions (which I call "acti-vators") signal when behavior can achieve a pleasant consequence (a reward) or avoid an unpleasant consequence (a penalty). Therefore, activators direct behavior, and consequences determine whether the behavior will recur. Accordingly, people are motivated by the consequences they expect to receive, escape, or avoid after perform-ing a target behavior.

Humanists maintain that this ABC (activator–behavior–consequence) analysis is much too simple to explain human behavior. For many applications, they are right. However, as shown in Figure 2.5 many of our daily behaviors are directed by pre-ceding activators and motivated by ensuing consequences. I have much more to say about this ABC approach to understanding and improving behavior in Parts 3 and 4 of this book. Then in Part 5, I explain how the person-based approach of the humanists can be integrated with the behavior-based approach to bring out the best in people and their organizations for the sake of achieving a Total Safety Culture.

Considering cost effectiveness

When people act in certain ways, they usually adjust their mental attitude and self-talk to parallel their actions; when people change their attitudes, values, or thinking strategies, certain behaviors change as a result. Thus, person-based and behavior-based approaches to changing people can influence both attitudes and behaviors, either directly or indirectly. Most parents, teachers, first-line supervisors, and safety managers use both approaches in their attempts to change a person's knowledge, skills, attitudes, or behaviors.

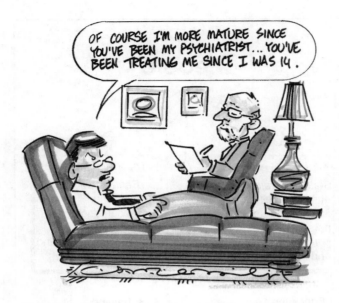

Figure 2.6 Psychotherapy can take a long time.

- When we lecture, counsel, or educate others in a one-on-one or group situation, we are essentially using a person-based approach.
- When we recognize, correct, or discipline others for what they have done, we are operating from a behavior-based perspective.

Unfortunately, we are not always effective with our person-based or behavior-based change techniques, and often we do not know whether our intervention worked as intended. In order to apply person-based techniques to psychotherapy, clinical psychologists receive specialized therapy or counseling training for four or more years, followed by an internship of at least one year. This intensive training is needed because tapping into an individual's perceptions, attitudes, and thinking styles is a demanding and complex process. Also, internal dimensions of people are extremely difficult to measure reliably, making it cumbersome to assess therapeutic progress and obtain straightforward feedback regarding therapy skills. Consequently, the person-based therapy process can be very time-consuming (see Figure 2.6), requiring numerous one-on-one sessions between professional therapist and client.

In contrast, behavior-based psychotherapy was designed to be administered by individuals with minimal professional training. From the start, the idea was to reach people where problems occur — in the home, school, rehabilitation institute, and workplace, for example — and teach parents, teachers, supervisors, friends, or coworkers the behavior-change techniques most likely to work under the circumstances.

More than three decades of research have shown convincingly that this on-site approach is cost effective, primarily because behavior-change techniques are straightforward and relatively easy to administer, and because intervention progress can be readily monitored by the ongoing observation of target behaviors. By obtaining

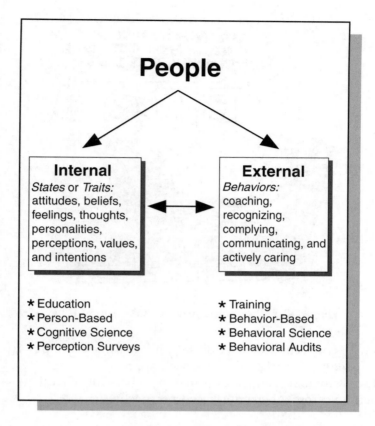

Figure 2.7 The internal and external aspects of people determine the success of a safety process.

objective feedback on the impact of intervention techniques, a behavior-based process can be continually refined.

Integrating approaches

A common perspective, even among psychologists, is that humanists and behaviorists are complete opposites. Behaviorists are considered cold, objective, and mechanistic, operating with minimal concern for people's feelings. In contrast, humanists are thought of as warm, subjective, and caring, with limited concern for *directly* changing another person's behavior or attitude.

Given the foundations of humanism and behaviorism, it is easy to build barriers between person-based and behavior-based perspectives and assume you must follow one or the other when designing an intervention process. In fact, many consultants in the safety management field market themselves as using one or the other approach, but not both. It is my firm belief that these approaches need to be integrated in order to truly understand the psychology of safety and build a Total Safety Culture.

In conclusion

Theory or basic principles are needed to organize research findings and guide our approaches to improve the safety and health of an organization. Similarly, a vision for a Total Safety Culture incorporated into a mission statement is needed to guide us in developing action plans to achieve safety excellence.

When employees understand and accept the mission statement and guiding principles, they become more involved in the mission. The action plan will not be viewed as one more flavor of the month, but as reflecting the right principles and useful for achieving shared goals. Indeed, the workforce will help design and implement the action plans. This is crucial for cultivating a Total Safety Culture.

A basic principle introduced in this chapter is that the safety performance of an organization results from the dynamic interaction of environment, behavior, and person factors. The behavior and person dimensions represent the human aspect of industrial safety and reflect two divergent approaches to understanding the psychology of injury prevention.

Figure 2.7 summarizes the distinction between person-based and behavior-based psychology and shows that both approaches contribute to understanding and helping people. Both the internal and external dimensions of people are covered in this book as they relate to improving organizational safety. Profound knowledge on the person side comes from cognitive science, whereas the behavior-based approach is founded on behavioral science.

The best I can do is provide education by improving your knowledge and thinking about the human dynamics of safety improvement. You will do the training by using the observation and feedback techniques detailed later in Part 4 to improve your own or someone else's behavior.

Taken alone, the behavior-based approach is more cost effective than the person-based approach in affecting large-scale change. But it cannot be effective unless the work culture believes in the behavior-based principles and willingly applies them to achieve the interdependent safety mission. This involves a person-based approach. Therefore, to achieve a Total Safety Culture we need to integrate person-based and behavior-based psychology. This text shows you how to meet this challenge.

chapter three

Paradigm shifts for total safety

This chapter outlines ten new perspectives we need to adopt in order to exceed current levels of safety excellence and reach our ultimate goal — a Total Safety Culture. The traditional three Es of safety management – engineering, education, and enforcement — have only gotten us so far. A Total Safety Culture requires understanding and applying three additional Es – empowerment, ergonomics, and evaluation.

"Mindsets are yesterday — mind growth is tomorrow." — Joe Batten

Safety in industry has improved dramatically in this century. Let's examine the evolution of accident prevention to see how this was accomplished. The first systematic research began in the early 1900s and focused on finding the psychological causes of accidents. It assumed people were responsible for most accidents and injuries, usually through mental errors caused by anxiety, attitude, fear, stress, personality, or emotional state. Reducing accidents was typically attempted by "readjusting" attitude or personality, usually through supervisor counseling or discipline.

This so-called "psychological approach" held that certain individuals were "accident prone." By removing these workers from risky jobs or by disciplining them to correct their attitude or personality problems, it was thought that accidents could be reduced. As I discussed in Chapter 1, this focus on accident proneness has not been effective, partly because reliable and valid measurement procedures are not available. Also, the person factors contributing to accident proneness are probably not consistent characteristics or traits within people, but vary from time to time and situation to situation.

The old three Es

Enthusiasm for the early "psychological approach" waned because of the difficulty in measuring its impact. In addition, the seminal research and scholarship of William Haddon (1968) suggested that engineering changes held the most promise for large-scale, long-term reductions in injury severity.

As the first administrator of the National Highway Safety Bureau [now the National Highway Traffic Safety Administration (NHTSA)], Dr. Haddon was able to turn his theory and research into the first federal automobile safety standards. Haddon believed injury is caused by delivering excess energy to the body, and that injury prevention depends on controlling that energy. The prevention focus now shifted to engineering and epidemiology, and resulted in developing personal protective equipment (PPE) for work and recreational environments, as well as standards and policy regarding the use of PPE. In vehicles, Haddon's basic theory eventually led to collapsible steering wheels, padded dashboards, head restraints, and air bags in automobiles.

This brief history of the safety movement in the United States explains why engineering is the dominant paradigm in industrial health and safety, with secondary emphasis on two additional "Es" – education and enforcement. Over the past several decades, the basic protocol for reducing injury has been to:

1. *Engineer* the safest equipment, environmental settings, and protective devices.
2. *Educate* people regarding the use of the engineering interventions.
3. Use discipline to *enforce* compliance with recommended safe work practices.

Thanks to this paradigm most safety professionals are safety *engineers* who commonly advocate that "Safety is a condition of employment."

The three Es have dramatically reduced injury severity in the workplace, at home, and on the road. Let's take a look at motor vehicle safety for a minute. The Government Accounting Office has estimated conservatively that the early automobile safety standards ushered through Congress by Haddon had saved at least 28,000 American lives by 1974. In addition, state laws passed in the 1980s requiring use of vehicle safety belts and child safety seats have saved countless more lives. Many *more* lives would be saved and injuries avoided if more people buckled up and used child safety seats for their children.

The current rate of safety belt use in the United States is about 70 percent, a dramatic improvement from the 15 percent prior to statewide interventions, including belt-use laws, campaigns to educate people about the value of safety-belt use, and large-scale enforcement blitzes by local and state police officers.

There is still much room for improvement, especially considering that most of the riskiest drivers still do not buckle up. Each year since 1990, the U.S. Department of Transportation has set nationwide belt-use goals of 70 percent, but to date this goal has not been met — at least over the long term. It seems the effectiveness of current methods to increase the use of this particular type of PPE has plateaued or asymptoted around 70 percent. Recently, President Clinton set the U.S. buckle-up goal at 85 percent by the year 2005. We just cannot get there with the same old intervention approaches.

Now, let's turn our attention to industry. I've worked with many corporate safety professionals over the years who say their plant's safety performance has reached a plateau. Yes, their overall safety record is vastly better than it once was, but continuous improvement is elusive. A frantic search for ways to take safety to the next level has not paid off. The old "three Es" paradigm will not get us there. A certain percentage of people keep falling through the cracks. Keep on doing what you're doing and you will keep on getting what you're getting. As I heard W. Edwards Deming (1991) say many times, "Goals without method: What could be worse?"

Three new Es

This book discusses the three new Es — ergonomics, empowerment, and evaluation. I certainly do not suggest abandoning tradition. We need to maintain a focus on engineering, education, and enforcement strategies. But to get beyond current plateaus and reach new heights in safety excellence, we must attend more competently to the psychology of injury prevention. These three new Es suggest specific directions or principles.

Ergonomics

As discussed in Chapter 1, *ergonomics* requires careful study of relationships between environment and behaviors, as well as developing action plans (such as equipment work orders, safer operating procedures, training exercises) to avoid possible acute or chronic injury from the environment–behavior interaction. This requires consistent and voluntary participation by those who perform the behaviors in the various work environments. These are usually line operators or hourly workers in an organization, and their participation will happen when these individuals are *empowered.* Throughout this book, I discuss ways to develop an empowered work culture and I explain procedures for involving employees in ergonomic interventions.

Empowerment

Some operational definitions of the traditional three Es for safety (especially *enforcement*) have been detrimental to employee empowerment. Many supervisors have translated "enforcement" into a strict punishment approach, and the result has turned off many employees to safety programs. These workers may do what is required, but no more. Some individuals who feel especially controlled by safety regulations might try to beat the system, and success will likely bring a sense of gratification or freedom, as illustrated in Figure 3.1.

I discuss this principle in more detail later, especially as it relates to developing behavior change interventions. At this point, I want you to understand that some types of enforcement are likely to inhibit empowerment and should be reconsidered and refined. Paradigms must change — the theme of this chapter.

Evaluation

The third new E word essential to achieving a Total Safety Culture is *evaluation.* Without appropriate feedback or evaluation, practice does not make perfect. Thus, we need the right kind of evaluation processes. Later in this book, especially Chapter 15, I detail procedures for conducting the right kind of comprehensive evaluation. Right now, what is important to understand is that some traditional methods of evaluation actually decrease or stifle empowerment. This calls for changing some safety measurement paradigms.

Remember the need for a guiding theory or set of principles? Basic theory from person-based and behavior-based psychology suggests shifts to new safety paradigms. These paradigm shifts provide a new set of guiding principles for achieving new heights in safety excellence.

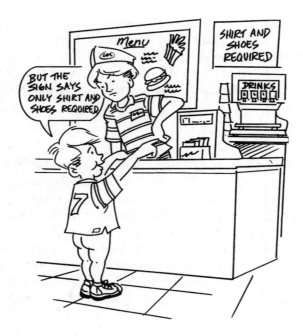

Figure 3.1 Some top-down rules have undesirable side effects.

Shifting paradigms

I want to define ten basic changes in belief, attitude, or perception that are needed to develop the ultimate Total Safety Culture. These shifts require new principles, approaches, or procedures, and will result in different behaviors and attitudes among top managers and hourly workers. Empowerment will increase throughout the work culture.

From government regulation to corporate responsibility

Many safety activities and programs in U.S. industry are driven by OSHA (the U.S. Occupational Safety and Health Administration) or MSHA (the Mine Safety and Health Administration) rather than by the employers and employees who can benefit from a safety process. In other words, many in industry do "safety stuff" because the government requires it — not because it was their idea and initiative.

People are more motivated and willing to go beyond the call of duty when they are achieving their own self-initiated goals. Ownership, commitment, and proactive behaviors are less likely when you are working to avoid missing goals or deadlines set by someone else. This statement is intuitive and reflected in Figure 3.2. Just compare your own motivation when working for personal gain vs. someone else's gain or when working to earn a reward vs. to avoid a penalty.

The language used to define safety programs and activities influences personal participation. Remember, we can act ourselves into an attitude. So it makes sense to talk about safety as a company mission that is owned and achieved by the very people

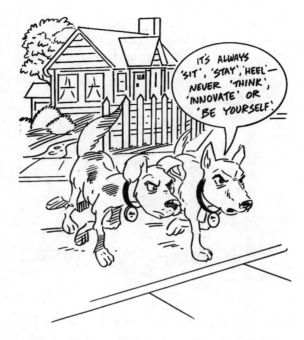

Figure 3.2 Top-down control stifles creativity.

it benefits. A safety process is not intended to benefit federal regulators. Let's work to achieve a Total Safety Culture for the right reasons.

From failure oriented to achievement oriented

If you strive to meet someone else's goals rather than your own, you will probably develop an attitude of "working to avoid failure" rather than "working to achieve success." We are more motivated by achieving success than avoiding failure. If you have a choice between earning positive reinforcers (rewards) or avoiding negative reinforcers (punishers), you will probably choose the positive reinforcement situation. Moreover, if you feel controlled by negative reinforcement, you often procrastinate and take a reactive rather than a proactive stance.

Figure 3.3 illustrates what I mean. The runner will surely start running, but how long will he run? When the coach is not around to threaten a negative consequence for not running, will he keep going? Will he practice on his own to improve his running skills? Will he hold himself accountable to be the best he can be on the running track? A "yes" answer to these questions will only occur if the runner can put himself in an achievement-oriented mindset. This is difficult in the enforcement context established by the coach.

This principle helps explain why more continuous and proactive attention goes to productivity and quality than to safety. Productivity and quality goals are typically stated in achievement terms, and gains are tracked and recorded as individual or team accomplishments, sometimes followed by rewards or recognition awards.

In contrast, safety goals are most often stated in negative reinforcement terms. How many times have you heard "we will reach our safety goal after another month

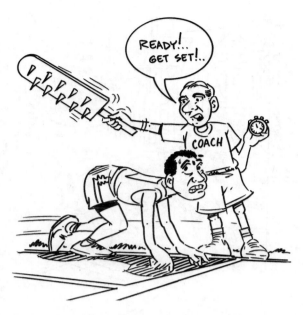

Figure 3.3 Working to avoid failure is not fun.

without a lost-time injury," and "keeping score" in safety means tracking and recording losses or injuries?

Measuring safety with only records of injuries not only limits evaluation to a reactive stance, but it also sets up a negative motivational system that is apt to take a back seat to the positive system used for productivity and quality. Giving safety an achievement perspective (like production and quality) requires a different scoring system, as indicated by the next paradigm shift.

From outcome focused to behavior focused

Companies are frequently ranked according to their OSHA recordables and lost-time injuries. Within companies, work groups or individual workers earn safety awards according to outcomes — those with the lowest numbers win. Offering incentives for fewer injuries, for instance, can often reduce the *reported* numbers while not improving safety. Pressure to reduce outcomes without changing the process (or ongoing behaviors) often causes employees to cover up their injuries.

How many times have you heard of an injured employee being driven to work each day to sign in and then promptly returned to the hospital or home to recuperate? This keeps the outcome numbers low, but does more harm than good to the corporate culture. Likewise, failure to report even a minor first-aid case prohibits key personnel from correcting the factors that led to the incident.

A misguided emphasis on outcomes rather than process is illustrated in Figure 3.4. Although the idea of a dead person receiving a safety reward is clearly ridiculous, this type of incentive/reward process is quite common in American industry. Such programs often bring down numbers by influencing the reporting of injuries, but rarely do they benefit the safety processes which control results.

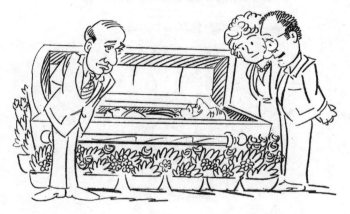

Figure 3.4 Safety reward programs should pass the "dead-man's test."

A scoring system based on what people do for safety not only attacks a contributing factor in most work injuries, it can also be achievement oriented. This puts safety in the same motivational framework as productivity and quality.

In Chapter 11, I explain principles for establishing an incentive/reward process to motivate the kinds of safety processes that influence outcomes. For now, just recognize and appreciate the advantage of focusing on achieving process improvements over working to avoid failure. This is especially true if a failure-oriented goal is remote, such as a plant-wide reduction in injuries, and thus might be perceived as uncontrollable.

Safety can be on equal footing with productivity and quality if it is recorded and tracked with an achievement score perceived by employees as directly controllable and attainable. This occurs with a focus on the safety processes that can decrease an organization's injury rate, as well as an ongoing measurement system that continuously tracks safety accomplishments and displays them to the workforce. This book shows you how to do this.

From top-down control to bottom-up involvement

As I discussed when introducing the three new Es, a Total Safety Culture requires continual involvement from operations personnel, such as hourly workers. After all, these are the people who know where safety hazards are located and when the at-risk behaviors occur. Also, they can have the most influence in supporting safe behaviors and correcting at-risk behaviors and conditions. In fact, the ongoing processes involved in developing a Total Safety Culture need to be supported from the top but driven from the bottom. This is more than employee participation; it's employee ownership, commitment, and empowerment.

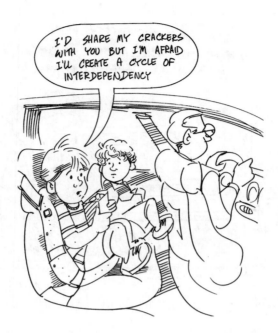

Figure 3.5 U.S. culture promotes more independence than interdependence.

From rugged individualism to interdependent teamwork

An employee-driven safety process requires teamwork founded on interpersonal trust, synergy, and win–win contingencies. However, from childhood most of us have been taught an individualistic, win–lose perspective, supported by such popular slogans as "You have to blow your own horn," "Nice guys finish last," "No one can fill your shoes like you," and "It's the squeaky wheel that gets the grease." Further-more, as shown in Figure 3.5, grades in school, the legal system, and many sports orient us to think win–lose independence rather than win–win interdependence. This is why a true team approach to safety does not come easily.

From a piecemeal to a systems approach

The long-term improvements of a Total Safety Culture can only be achieved with a systems approach, including balanced attention to all aspects of the corporate cul-ture. Deming (1986b, 1993) emphasized that total quality only can be achieved through a systems approach, and of course the same is true for safety. As I discussed in Chapter 2, three basic domains need attention when designing and evaluating safety processes and when investigating the root causes of near hits and injuries:

1. *Environment* factors such as equipment, tools, machines, housekeeping, heat/cold, and engineering
2. *Person* factors such as employees' knowledge, skills, abilities, intelligence, mo-tives, and personality
3. *Behavior* factors such as complying, coaching, recognizing, communicating, and "actively caring"

Two of these system variables involve human factors. Each generally receives less attention than the environment, mostly because it is more difficult to visibly measure the outcomes of efforts to change the human factors. Some human factors programs focus on behaviors (as in behavior-based safety); others focus on attitudes (as in a person-based approach). A Total Safety Culture integrates these two approaches.

From fault finding to fact finding

Blaming an individual or group of individuals for an injury-producing incident is not consistent with a systems approach to safety. Instead, an injury or near hit provides an opportunity to gather facts from all aspects of the system that could have contributed to the incident. However, most evaluations of near hits or injuries are incomplete, and are much less informative than they could be. Part of the problem here is the very term we use to describe the process — *accident investigation.*

Accident investigation is a common phrase in industrial safety and health, but what does it mean? It actually implies "a chance occurrence" outside your immediate control. When a child has an "accident" in his pants, we presume he was not in control. He could not help it.

And what about the word "investigation"? Doesn't this term imply a hunt for some single cause or person to blame for a particular incident, as in "criminal investigation"? How can we promote fact-finding over fault-finding with a term like "investigation" defining our job assignment?

Truly, to learn more about how to prevent injuries from an analysis of an incident, we need to approach the task with a different mindset. It's not "accident investigation" — it's "incident analysis." This simple substitution of words can have great impact. We can get more employee participation in the process and reap more benefits.

From reactive to proactive

Analyzing events preceding an incident, be it a near hit or an injury, demonstrates the need to think and act proactively. Unfortunately, a proactive stance is extremely difficult to maintain, especially in a corporate culture that is increasingly complex and demanding. There is a higher and higher price tag on "free time." With barely enough time to react sufficiently to crises each day, how can we find time to be proactive?

Proactivity is especially challenging within the context of downsizing, disguised as "re-engineering" in many work cultures. The worker in Figure 3.6 is barely able to react effectively to daily crises. How can he be expected to think ahead and be proactive? There are no quick-fix answers, but injury prevention requires us to find solutions. This text provides theory, procedures, and tools to guide long-term continuous improvement. Thus, we need to accept the next paradigm shift.

From quick fix to continuous improvement

"Proactive" can be substituted for "reactive" only with a systems perspective and an optimistic attitude of continuous improvement through increased employee involvement. Understanding the psychology of safety can be a great aid here. The principles and procedures described in this book will enable you to influence incremental changes in work practices and attitudes that can prevent an injury. This represents a

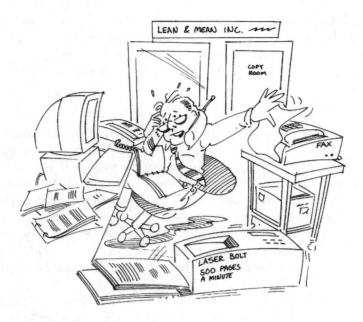

Figure 3.6 Technology cannot always substitute for personnel.

proactive, continuous improvement paradigm, which will surely improve your safety performance.

From priority to value

"Safety is a priority." This is probably the most common safety slogan found in workplaces and voiced by safety leaders. I have seen signs, pens, buttons, hats, T-shirts, and notepads with this message. No wonder safety and health professionals are surprised when I say that safety should *not* be a priority. To justify my case, I offer the following explanation.

Think about a typical workday morning. We all follow a prioritized agenda, often a standard routine, before traveling to work. Some people eat a hearty breakfast, read the morning newspaper, take a shower, and wash dishes. Others wake up early enough to go for a morning jog before work. Some grab a roll and a cup of coffee, and leave their home in disarray until they get back in the evening.

In each of these scenarios the agendas — the priorities — are different. Yet, there is one common activity. It's not a priority but a basic value. Do you know what it is?

One morning you wake up late. Perhaps your alarm clock failed. You have only 15 minutes to prepare for work. Your morning routine changes drastically. Priorities must be rearranged. You might skip breakfast, a shower, or a shave. Yet every morning schedule still has one item in common. It's not a priority, capable of being dropped from a routine due to time constraints or a new agenda. No, this particular morning activity represents a *value* which we've been taught as infants, and it's never compromised. Have you guessed it by now? Yes, this common link in everyone's morning routine, regardless of time constraints, is "getting dressed."

This simple scenario shows how circumstances can alter behavior and priorities. Actually, labeling a behavior a "priority" implies that its order in a hierarchy of daily activities can be rearranged. How often does this happen at work? Does safety sometimes take a "back seat" when the emphasis is on other priorities such as production quantity or quality?

Enduring values

It's human nature to shift priorities, or behavioral hierarchies, according to situational demands or contingencies. But values remain constant. The early morning anecdote illustrates that the activity of "getting dressed" is a value that is never dropped from the routine. Should "working safely" not hold the same status as "getting dressed"? Safe work practices should occur regardless of the demands of a particular day.

Safety should be a value linked with every activity or priority in a work routine. Safe work should be the enduring norm, whether the current focus is on quantity, quality, or cost effectiveness as the "number one priority."

The ultimate aim of a Total Safety Culture is to make safety an integral aspect of all performance, regardless of the task. Safety should be more than the behaviors of "using personal protective equipment," more than "locking out power" and "checking equipment for potential hazards," and more than "practicing good housekeeping." Safety should be an unwritten rule, a social norm, that workers follow regardless of the situation. It should become a value that is never questioned — never compromised.

In conclusion

This chapter describes ten shifts in perspective needed to go beyond current levels of safety excellence. The first nine could be considered goals for achieving a Total Safety Culture. The tenth — making safety a value — is not something that can be measured and tracked. It's the ideal vision for our safety mission.

Here is how the new paradigms fit together. Your safety achievement process should be considered a company responsibility, not a regulatory obligation. It should be achievement oriented with a focus on behaviors, supported by all managers and supervisors but driven by the line workers or operators through interdependent teamwork. A systems approach is needed, which leads to a fact-finding perspective, a proactive stance, and a commitment to continuous improvement.

These new perspectives reflect new principles to follow, new procedures to develop and implement. This "new safety work" will lead to different perceptions, attitudes, and even values. Ultimately, the tenth paradigm shift can be reached. When safety goes from priority to value, it will not be compromised at work, at home, or on the road. Naturally, numerous injuries will be prevented and lives saved every day. This vision should motivate each of us to be active in the safety achievement process. This book helps you define your role.

part two

Human barriers to safety

chapter four

The complexity of people

Safety is usually a continuous fight with human nature. This chapter explains why. Understanding this basic point will lead to less victim blaming and fault finding when analyzing an injury. Instead, we will be able to find factors in the system that can be changed in advance to prevent injuries at work, at home, and throughout the community.

"What lies behind us and what lies before us are small matters compared to what lies within us." — Ralph Waldo Emerson

"All injuries are preventable."
"It's human nature to work safely."
"Safety is just common sense."
"Safety is a condition of employment."

Read these familiar statements and you get the idea that working safely is easy or natural. Nothing could be farther from the truth.

In fact, it's often more convenient, more comfortable, more expedient, and more common to take risks than to work safely. And past experience usually supports our decisions to choose the at-risk behavior, whether we are working, traveling, or playing. So, we are often engaged in a continuous fight with human nature to motivate ourselves and others to avoid those risky behaviors and maintain safe ones.

Let's consider what holds us back from choosing the safe way, whether it's following safe operating procedures, driving our automobiles, or using personal protective equipment.

Fighting human nature

When I ask safety professionals, corporate executives, or hourly workers what causes work-related injuries, I get long and varied lists of factors. Actually, each list is quite similar. After all, everyone experiences events, attitudes, demands, distractions, responsibilities, and circumstances that get in the way of performing a task safely.

Most of us have been in situations where we were not sure how to perform safely. Perhaps we lacked training. Maybe the surrounding environment was not as safe as it could be. Demands from a supervisor, coworker, or friend put pressure on us to take a short cut or risk. Maybe, it was inconvenient or uncomfortable to follow all of the safety procedures. It's possible our physical condition — fatigue, boredom, drug impairment — influenced at-risk performance.

There are other factors. Have you ever been unsafely distracted by external stimuli, like another person's presence or by an internal state, like personal thoughts or emotions? Can you remember a time when you just did not feel like taking the extra time to be safe? I am sure you have experienced the "macho" attitude, from yourself or others that "It will never happen to me." Fortunately, it's rare that an injury follows unsafe behavior. The attitude "It won't happen to me" is usually supported or rewarded by our actual experiences. Risk taking is rarely punished with an injury or even a near hit, instead it is consistently rewarded with convenience, comfort, or time saved.

This creates something of a vicious cycle. The rewards of risky behavior mean you are likely to take more chances. As you gain experience at work you often master dangerous shortcuts. Because these at-risk behaviors are not followed by a near hit or injury, they remain unpunished, and they persist.

This basic principle of human nature reinforced throughout our lives runs counter to the safety efforts of individuals, groups, organizations, and communities. It explains why promoting safety and health is a most difficult and ongoing challenge at work. The reality is that injuries really do happen to the "other guy."

Dimensions of human nature

The factors contributing to a work injury can be categorized into three areas:

1. Environment factors
2. Person factors
3. Behavior factors

This is the "Safety Triad" introduced in Chapter 2. The most common reaction to an injury is to correct something about the environment — modify or fix equipment, tools, housekeeping, or an environmental hazard.

Often the incident report includes some mention of person factors, like the employee's knowledge, skills, ability, intelligence, motives, or personality. These factors are typically translated into general recommendations:

"The employee will be disciplined."
"The employee will be retrained."

This kind of vague attention to critical human aspects of a work injury shows how frustrating and difficult it is to deal with the psychology of safety — the person and behavior sides of the Safety Triad. The human factors contributing to injury are indeed complex, often unpredictable and uncontrollable. This justifies my conclusion that all injuries cannot be prevented.

The acronym BASIC ID reflects the complexity and uncontrollability of human nature. As depicted in Figure 4.1, each letter represents one of seven human dimensions of an individual. Here's a simple scenario that underscores the need in safety to understand various human factors.

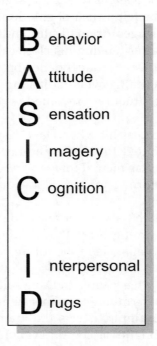

B ehavior
A ttitude
S ensation
I magery
C ognition
I nterpersonal
D rugs

Figure 4.1   The acronym BASIC ID reflects the complexity of people
and potential contributions to injury.

Dave, an experienced and skilled craftsman, works rapidly to make an equipment adjustment while the machinery continues to operate. As he works, production-line employees watch and wait to resume their work. Dave realizes all too well that the sooner he finishes his task, the sooner his coworkers can resume quality production. So, he does not shut down and lock out the equipment power. After all, he has adjusted this equipment numerous times before without locking out and he has never gotten injured.

A morning argument with his teenage daughter pervades Dave's thoughts as he works, and suddenly he experiences a near hit. His late timing nearly results in his hand being crushed in a pinch point.

Removing his hand just in time, Dave feels weak in his knees and begins to perspire. This stress reaction is accompanied by a vivid image of a crushed right hand. After gathering his composure, Dave walks to the switch panel, shuts down and locks out the power, then lights up a cigarette. He thinks about this scary event for the rest of the day and talks about the near hit to fellow workers during his breaks.

This brief episode illustrates each of the psychological dimensions represented by BASIC ID (see Figure 4.1) and demonstrates the complexity of human activity.

Behavior is illustrated by observable actions such as adjusting equipment, pulling a hand away from the moving machinery, lighting up a cigarette, and talking to coworkers.

Dave's **attitude** about work was fairly neutral at the start of the day, but immediately following his near hit he felt a rush of emotion. His attitude toward "energy control and power lockout" changed dramatically, and his commitment to following lockout procedures increased after relating his close call to friends.

Sensation is evidenced by Dave's dependence on visual acuity, hand–eye coordination, and a keen sense of timing when adjusting the machinery. His ability to react quickly to the dangerous situation prevented severe pain and potential loss of valuable touch sensation.

Imagery occurred after the near hit when Dave visualized a crushed hand in his "mind's eye," and this contributed to the significance and distress of the incident. Dave will probably experience this mental image periodically for some time to come. This will motivate him to perform appropriate lockout procedures, at least for the immediate future.

Cognition or "mental speech" about the morning argument with his daughter may have contributed to the timing error that resulted in the near hit. Dave will probably remind himself of this episode in the future, and these cognitions may help trigger proper lockout behavior.

Interpersonal refers to the other people in Dave's life who contributed to his near hit and will be influential in determining whether he initiates and maintains appropriate lockout practices. For example, it was the interpersonal discussion with his daughter that occupied his thoughts or cognitions before the near hit. The presence of production-line workers influenced Dave through subtle peer pressure to quickly adjust equipment without lockout practices. These onlookers may have distracted Dave from the task, or they could have motivated him to show off his adjustment skills. After Dave's near hit, his interpersonal discussions were therapeutic, helping him relieve his distress and increase his personal commitment to occupational safety.

Drugs in the form of caffeine from morning coffee may have contributed to Dave's timing error. The extra cigarettes Dave smoked as a "natural" reaction to distress also had physiological consequences, which could have been reflected in Dave's subsequent behavior, attitude, sensation, or cognition.

Dave's lesson shows how human nature interacts with environmental factors to cause at-risk work practices, near hits, and sometimes personal injuries. It's relatively easy to control the environmental factors. As I explain in Part 3 on behavior-based safety, it's feasible to measure and control the behavior factors. However, the complex person factors, described by the BASIC ID acronym, are quite elusive. The field of psychology provides insights here, and this information can benefit occupational safety and health programs.

Let's further discuss aspects of human nature that can make safety achievement so challenging.

Cognitive failures

"All injuries are preventable." I have heard this said so many times that it seems to be a slogan or personal affirmation that safety pros use to keep themselves motivated. I suspect some readers will resist any challenge to this ideal. I certainly appreciate their optimism, and there is no harm if such perfectionism is kept to oneself. But sharing this belief with others can actually inhibit achieving a Total Safety Culture.

You see, if a common workplace slogan declares all injuries preventable, workers may be reluctant to admit they were injured or had a near hit. After all, if *all* injuries are preventable and I have an injury, I must be a real "jerk" for getting hurt.

Combine this slogan with a *goal* of zero injuries and a *reward* for not having an injury and human nature will dictate covering up an injury if possible. Also, as I discuss in the next chapter, claiming that all injuries are preventable can reduce the perceived risk of the situation. This can create the notion that "it will not happen to me," a perception that can increase the probability of at-risk behavior and an eventual injury.

Eliminate the "all injuries are preventable" slogan from your safety discussions. The most important reason to drop it is that most people do not believe it anyway. They have been in situations where all the factors contributing to the near hit or injury could not have been anticipated, controlled, or prevented. The most uncontrollable factors are the person-based or internal subjective dimensions of people. Consider, for example, the role of cognitive failures. Donald Norman (1988) classifies various types of cognitive failure according to a particular stage of routine thinking and decision making. More specifically, consider that we continually take in, process, and react to information in our surroundings. Almost everything we do results from this basic information processing cycle.

We sense a stimulus (input), we evaluate the stimulus and plan a course of action (interpretation and decision making), and then we execute a response (output). Unintentional cognitive errors usually occur at the input and output stage of information processing. Judgment errors and calculated risks occur at the middle cognitive stage — interpretation and decision making.

Capture errors

Have you ever started traveling in one direction (like to the store) but suddenly find yourself on a more familiar route (like on the way to work)? How many times have you borrowed someone's pen to write a note or sign a form, and later found the pen in your pocket? Norman calls these "capture errors," because a familiar activity or routine seemingly "captures" you and takes over an unfamiliar activity. This error seems to occur at the execution stage of information processing, but it also involves misperception or inattention to relevant stimuli, as well as the absence of conscious judgment or decision making.

How does this error slip into the work routine? Have you ever started a new task and found yourself using old habits? Has a change in personal protective equipment (PPE) requirements influenced this kind of human error? It seems reasonable that a routine way of doing something (even at home) could "capture" your execution of a new work process and lead to this type of cognitive failure and an injury.

Description errors

These "brain cramps" occur when the descriptions or locators of the correct (safe) and incorrect (at-risk) executions are similar. For example, I periodically throw a tissue in our clothes hamper instead of the waste can, even though our clothes hamper is not next to a trash receptacle. On a few occasions, I have actually thrown dirty clothes in the trash can, and once I threw a sweaty T-shirt in the toilet. According to

Norman, the similar characteristic of these three items — a large oval opening — led to these errors.

Do you have any switches in your work setting which are similar and nearby but control different functions? How unsafe would it be to throw the wrong switch? Many control panels are designed with this error in mind. Switches or knobs controlling incompatible functions are not located in close proximity with one another and often look and feel distinctly different for quick visual and tactile discrimination. Thus, it might be useful to evaluate your work setting with regard to the need for different behaviors with similar descriptions.

Loss-of-activation errors

Have you ever walked into a room to do something or to get a certain object, but when you got there you forgot what you were there for? You think hard but just cannot remember. Then, you go back to the first room and suddenly you remember what you wanted to do or get in the other room. What happened here?

This cognitive failure is commonly referred to as "forgetting." Dr. Norman refers to it as "loss of activation," because the cue or activator that got the behavior started was lost or forgotten. This happens whenever you start an activity with a clear and specific goal, but after you get engaged in the task you lose sight of the goal. You might, in fact, continue the task but with little awareness of the rationale for progress toward a goal.

When people tell you they already know what to do with statements like "Stop harping on the same old thing," you can say you are just actively caring by trying to prevent a "loss-of-activation" error. You will never know how many of these cognitive failures you will prevent, but you can motivate yourself to keep activating by reflecting on your own experiences with this sort of "brain cramp." Then, consider the large number of people in your work setting who make similar unintentional errors every day.

Mode errors

Mode errors are probable whenever we face a task involving multiple options or modes of operation. These errors are inevitable when equipment is designed to have more functions than the number of control switches available. In other words, when controls are designed for more than one mode of operation, you can expect occurrences of this error.

Over the years, I have owned a variety of digital watches with a stopwatch mode. Each one has had a different arrangement of switches designed to provide more functions than control buttons. Therefore, the meaning of a button press depends upon the position of a mode switch. So, guess how many times I have pressed the wrong button and illuminated the dial or reset the digital readout when I only wanted to stop the timer? Have you experienced the same kind of mode error, if not with a stop watch, perhaps with the text editor of a personal computer? Airline pilots must be especially wary of this kind of error.

Mistakes and calculated risks

The four types of cognitive failures discussed so far — capture, description, loss-of-activation, and mode errors — are unintentional. Their sources are mostly at the input and output stages of information processing. The middle interpretation and decision-making stage is essentially uninvolved. Thus, the at-risk behavior resulting from these errors is unintentional. The person meant well. The plan was good, but the execution was unintentionally flawed.

Mistakes and calculated risks occur at the interpretation and decision-making stage of information processing. Here is where we interpret our sensory input and decide on a course of action. With mistakes, the individual was well-intentioned regarding the ultimate outcome of getting the job done, but used poor judgment in getting there.

While driving, have you ever turned right on to a main road into the path of an oncoming vehicle you had not seen, or whose speed you had misjudged? Have you ever miscalculated a parking space and scraped an adjoining vehicle? How many times have you planned a bad travel route and got caught in traffic congestion you could have avoided? Have you ever pressed the brake too quickly on a slippery road or pumped the brakes in an antilock system? Parking and braking are frequent and intentional driving behaviors, but under certain circumstances they are mistakes.

Now suppose you do not buckle your safety belt. Perhaps you divide your attention between the road and some other task like map reading, phone dialing, or cassette selecting. You know this behavior is unsafe, but you decide to take a calculated risk. Your judgment is faulty, as in a mistake, but unlike a mistake, your at-risk behavior is deliberate. Such behavior might seem rational because it is not followed by a negative consequence, and it is supported with perceived comfort, convenience, or efficiency.

Interpersonal factors

Our interpersonal relationships dramatically influence our thoughts, attitudes, and actions. How much of your time each day is dedicated to gaining the approval of others? Of course, we sometimes attempt to avoid the disapproval of others, be they a parent, spouse, work supervisor, or department head. As discussed in Chapter 3, we do not feel as good — or as "free" — when working to avoid failure or disapproval as when working to achieve success or approval. In both cases, other people are the cause of our motivation and behavior.

Is the scenario depicted in Figure 4.2 completely ridiculous and unrealistic? Well, it is a bit extreme, but consider for a moment the adversity many people go through to impress others. And have you ever followed orders you know put yourself or others at some degree of risk? If something went wrong, it would not be your fault. It was not your responsibility; you were just following orders. Just like when we were kids and we got into trouble, we were quick to say, "It's not my fault, he told me to do it."

It's not hard to see what all of this has to do with safety in the workplace. People take risks on the job because others do the same, and sometimes workers blindly follow a supervisor's orders that could endanger them, other coworkers, or the environment. This reflects the interpersonal power of two principles of social influence —

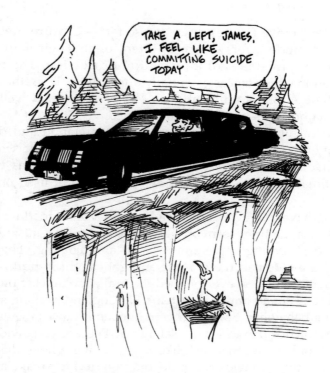

Figure 4.2 Authority can be taken too far.

conformity and authority. Let's examine these interpersonal phenomena more closely to understand exactly how they can be human barriers to safety. Then we can consider ways to turn these social influence factors around and use them to benefit safety.

Peer influence

The phenomenon of social conformity, depicted humorously in Figure 4.3, is certainly not new to any reader. We see examples of it every day, from the clothes people wear, to how they communicate both verbally and in writing. We cannot overlook the power of conformity in influencing at-risk behavior. We have learned that peer pressure increases when more people are involved and when the group members are seen as relatively competent or experienced.

It's important to remember, though, that one dissenter — a leader willing to ignore peer pressure and do the right thing — is often enough to prevent another person from succumbing to potentially dangerous conformity at work.

Power of authority

Imagine you are among nearly 1000 participants in one of Stanley Milgram's 20 obedience studies at Yale University in the 1960s. You and another individual are led to a laboratory to participate in a human learning experiment. First, you draw slips of paper out of a hat to determine randomly who will be the "teacher" and the "learner."

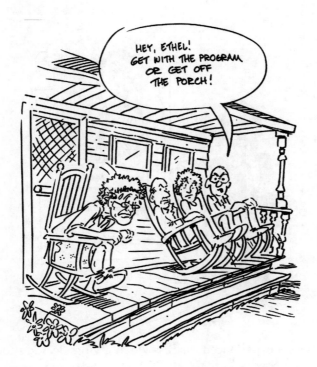

Figure 4.3 Peer pressure drives social conformity.

You get to be the teacher; the learner is taken to an adjacent room and strapped to a chair wired through the wall to an electric shock machine containing 30 switches with labels ranging from 15 volts — light shock to 450 volts — severe shock. You sit behind this shock generator and are instructed to punish the learner for errors in the learning task by delivering brief electric shocks, starting with the 15-volt switch and moving up to the next higher voltage with each of the learner's errors. The scenario is depicted in Figure 4.4.

Complying with the experimenter's instructions, you hear the learner moan as you flick the third, fourth, and fifth switches. When you flick the eighth switch (labeled 120 volts), the learner screams, "These shocks are painful," and when the tenth switch is activated, the learner shouts, "Get me out of here!"

At this point, you might think about stopping, but the experimenter prompts you with words like, "Please continue — the experiment requires that you continue."

Increasing the shock intensity with each of the learner's errors, you reach the 330-volt level. Now you hear shrieks of pain — the learner pounds on the wall, then becomes silent. Still, the experimenter urges you to flick the 450-volt switch when the learner fails to respond to the next question.

At what point will you refuse to obey the instructions?

Milgram asked this question of a group of people, including 40 psychiatrists, before conducting the experiment. They thought the sadistic game would stop soon after the learner indicated the shock was painful. So Milgram and his associates (1963) were surprised that 65 percent of his subjects, ranging in age from 20 to 50, went along with the experimenter's request right up to the last 450-volt switch.

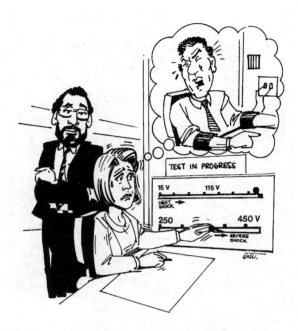

Figure 4.4 Subjects experienced distress when giving electric shocks to peers.

Why did they keep following along? Did they figure out the learner was a con-federate of the experimenter and did not really receive the shocks? Did they realize they were being deceived in order to test their obedience?

No, the subjects sweated, trembled, and bit their lips when giving the shocks, as shown in Figure 4.4. Some laughed nervously. Others openly questioned the instruc-tions, but most did as they were told.

Milgram and associates learned more about the power of authority in further studies. Full obedience exceeded 65 percent, with as many as 93 percent flicking the highest shock switch, when

- The authority figure — the one giving the orders — was in the room with the subject.
- The authority was supported by a prestigious institution, such as Yale Univer-sity.
- The shocks were given by a group of "teachers" in disguise and remaining anonymous.
- There was no evidence of resistance — no other subject was observed disobeying the experimenter.
- The victim was depersonalized or distanced from the subject in another room.

Milgram drew this lesson from the research: "Ordinary people, simply doing their jobs and without any particular hostility on their part, can become agents in a terrible destructive process" (Milgram, 1974).

Let's apply this research to the workplace. As a result of social obedience or social conformity, people might perform risky acts or overlook obvious safety hazards, and

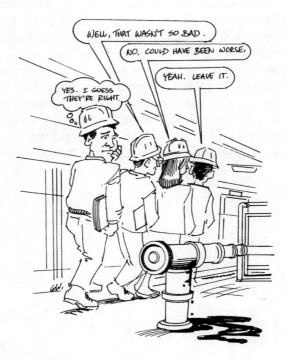

Figure 4.5 Social conformity and obedience can inhibit safety-related behavior.

put themselves and others in danger. To say "I was just following orders" reflects the obedience phenomenon, and "Everyone else does it!" implies social conformity or peer pressure.

To achieve a Total Safety Culture, we need to realize the power of these two interpersonal factors. Interventions capable of overcoming peer pressure and blind obedience are detailed in Part 4 of this book. What I want to stress at this point is the vital role of leadership. One person can make a difference — decreasing both destructive conformity and obedience — by deviating from the norm and setting a safe example. And when a critical mass of individuals boards the "safety bandwagon," you get constructive conformity and obedience that support a Total Safety Culture.

In conclusion

We need to understand a problem as completely as possible and from many perspectives before we can solve it. In this chapter, we explored dimensions of the safety problem by considering the complexity of people. I attempted to convince you that human nature does not usually support safety. The natural relationships between behavior and its motivating consequences usually result in some form of convenient, time-saving — and risky — behavior. Consequently, to achieve a Total Safety Culture, you should prepare for an ongoing fight with human nature.

Human barriers to safety are represented by a popular acronym from clinical psychology (BASIC ID). The "C" (cognitions) and second "I" (interpersonal) dimensions of this acronym, in particular, explain the special challenges of achieving a Total

Safety Culture. The phenomenon of cognitive failures shows the shallowness — in fact, the potential danger — of the popular safety slogan "All injuries are preventable." Conformity and obedience, two powerful phenomena from social psychological research, further help us understand the individual, group, and system factors responsible for at-risk behavior and injury. Both of these social phenomena influence the kind of at-risk behavior depicted in Figure 4.5.

The human barriers to safety discussed here should lead us to be more defensive and alert in hazardous environments. They also show how difficult it is to find the factors contributing to a near hit or injury. Another psychological challenge to safety is explored in the next chapter when we discuss the "S" (sensation) of BASIC ID.

chapter five

Sensation, perception, and perceived risk

It is critically important to understand that perceptions of risk vary among individuals. We cannot dramatically improve safety until people increase their perception of risk in various situations and reduce their overall tolerance for risk.

In this chapter we explore the notion of selective sensation or perception, and then relate this concept to perceived risk and injury control. Several factors are discussed that impact whether employees react to workplace hazards with alarm, apathy, or something in between. Taken together, these factors shape personal perceptions of risk and illustrate why the job of improving safety is so challenging.

"What we see depends mainly on what we look for." — John Lubbock

The "S" of the BASIC ID acronym introduced in Chapter 4 refers to **sensation** — a human dimension that influences our thinking, attitudes, emotions, and behavior. In grade school, we learned there are five basic senses we use daily to experience our world (we see, hear, smell, taste, and touch). Later we learned that our senses do not take in all of the information available in our immediate surroundings. Instead, we intentionally and unintentionally tune in and tune out certain features of our environment; thus, some potential experiences are never realized.

Selective sensation or perception

At the 1994 Professional Development Conference of the American Society of Safety Engineers (ASSE), the following instructions were printed in one-half of the 40-page handouts distributed to the audience of more than 350 individuals at the start of my two-hour presentation.

> You are going to look briefly at a picture and then answer some questions about it. The picture is a rough sketch of a poster of a couple at a costume ball. Do not dwell on the picture. Look at it only long enough to "take it all in" at once. After this, you will answer "yes" or "no" to a series of questions.

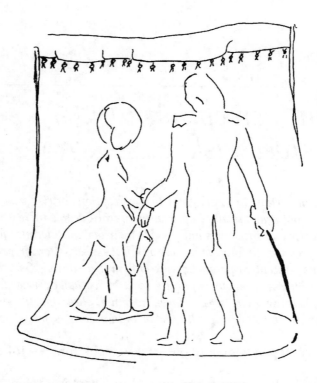

Figure 5.1 Selective sensation can be demonstrated with this ambiguous drawing.

After the participants read the instructions, I presented the illustration depicted in Figure 5.1 for about five seconds. If you would like to experience the biased visual sensation (or perception) demonstrated to the ASSE audience, please read the instructions previously given and then look at Figure 5.1 for approximately five seconds. Then, answer the questions that I asked my ASSE audience.

1. Did you see a man in the picture?
2. Did you see a woman in the picture?
3. Did you see an animal in the picture? If so, what kind of animal did you see? What other details did you detect in the brief exposure to the drawing?

    ___ A woman's purse?
    ___ A man's cane?
    ___ A trainer's whip?
    ___ A fish?
    ___ A ball?
    ___ A curtain?
    ___ A test?

Practically everyone in the audience raised a hand to answer "yes" to the first question, and I suspect you also see a man in Figure 5.1. But only about one-half of the audience acknowledged seeing a woman in the drawing, and many said they had seen an animal. When I asked what type of animal, the common response heard across the room was "seal." This drew many laughs, and the laughter got louder when I asked what else was quickly perceived in the illustration.

Several people saw a woman's purse and a man's cane; others said they had seen a trainer's whip, a fish, and a beach ball. Some remembered seeing a curtain. Others saw part of a circus tent. What did you see in Figure 5.1?

"What's going on here?" I asked the ASSE audience. Why are we getting these diverse reactions to one simple picture? Some people speculated about environmental factors in the seminar room, including lighting, spatial orientation, and visual distance from the presentation screen. Others thought individual differences, including gender, age, occupation, and personal experiences "last night" could be responsible. Finally, someone asked whether the instructions printed in their handouts could have influenced the different perceptions. This was, in fact, the case.

Every handout included the same exact instructions except for a few words. Included in one-half were all the words given above; the rest had the words "trained seal act" substituted for "couple at a costume ball." This was enough to make a marked difference in perceptions. Perhaps, this makes perfect sense to you. Critical words in the instructions created expectations for a particular visual experience. I had set up my audience. Was your perception of Figure 5.1 influenced by this "set up"?

Biased by context

Take a look at Figure 5.2. I suspect you have no difficulty reading the sentence as "The cat sat by the door," even though the symbol for "H" is exactly the same as the symbol for "A." It is a matter of context. The symbol was positioned in a way that influenced your labeling (or encoding) of the symbol. Likewise, the context or environmental surroundings in our visual field influence how we see particular stimuli.

The same is true for our other senses — hearing, smelling, tasting, and touching. How we experience food, which involves the sensations of smell, touch, and taste, can be dramatically influenced by the atmosphere in which it is served. This is a basic rule of the restaurant business. Of course, other factors also bias food sensations, including hunger and past experiences with the same and similar food.

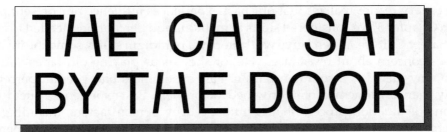

Figure 5.2 The context or circumstances surrounding a stimulus can influence how we perceive it.

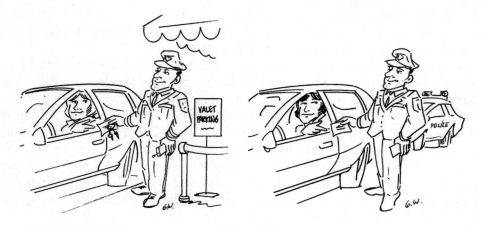

Figure 5.3 The environment context influences personal perception
of the man in uniform.

Now take a look at Figure 5.3. What label do you give the man in the drawing on the left? The setting or context certainly influences your decision. The sign, keys, and uniform are cues that the man is probably a doorman. The environmental context in the drawing on the right leads to a different perception and label for the same person. Here, he is a policeman enforcing a safety policy.

Now let us take our discussion of perception and apply it to the workplace. Here, perceptions of people can be shaped by equipment, housekeeping, job titles, and work attire. In fact, our own job title or work assignment can influence our perceptions of ourselves, as well as affect our perceptions of others. This can dramatically influence how we interact with others if, indeed, we choose to interact at all.

It is important to recognize this contextual bias. Pick out someone you communicate with at work, and think how your relationship would be different in another setting. Would you still feel superior or inferior? The work setting has a way of turning individuals into numbers, depersonalizing them. This impression certainly can be misleading and might cause you to overlook someone's potential. In another setting, the same individual might feel empowered and be perceived as a leader.

Biased by our past

Perhaps every reader realizes that our past experiences influence our present perceptions. In Chapter 3, we considered shifts in methods and perceptions needed to achieve a Total Safety Culture. When I give workshops on paradigm shifts, someone invariably expresses concern about resistance. "He (or she) keeps playing old tapes and is not open to new ideas" is a common refrain. Past experiences bias present perceptions. Actually, there is a long trail of intertwined factors here. Past experiences filter through a personal evaluation process that is influenced by person factors, including many past perceived experiences. The cumulative collection of these previous perceived experiences biases every new experience and makes it indeed difficult to "teach an old dog new tricks."

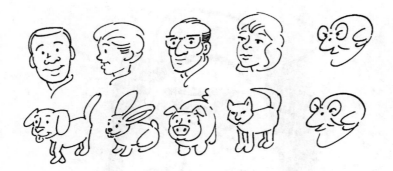

Figure 5.4 Prior perceptual experience influences current perception.
Adapted from Bugelski and Alimpay (1961).

Some participants arrive at my seminars and workshops with a "closed mind" and a "have to be here" attitude. Others start with an "open mind" and an "opportunity to learn" outlook. This is another example of the power of personal perception — how much one learns at these seminars depends on perceptions.

Perhaps you will find it worthwhile to copy Figure 5.4 and use it for a group demonstration. You can show how current impressions are affected by prior perceptions by asking participants to call out what they see as you reveal each drawing. The drawings must be uncovered in a particular order. Show the top row of pictures first, revealing each successive one from left to right. The last picture will probably be identified as the face of an elderly man.

With the top row covered, show the successive animal pictures of the second row. Now, the last picture will likely be identified as a rat or mouse. Even after knowing the purpose of the demonstration, you can view serially the row pictures in Figure 5.4 and see how your perception of the last drawing changes depending on whether you previously looked at human faces or animals.

Now, take a look at the woman in Figure 5.5. Notice anything strange, other than the picture is upside down? Is this face relatively attractive, or at least normal? Now turn the book upside down and view the woman's face from the normal orientation. Has your perception changed? Why did you not notice her awkward (actually ugly) mouth when the picture was upside down? Perhaps both context and prior experience (or learning) biased your initial perception. I bet this perceptual bias will persist even after you realize the cause of the distortion, and after viewing the face several times in both positions. A biased perception can be difficult to correct. It's not easy to fight human nature.

Relevance to achieving a Total Safety Culture

Is the relevance of this discussion to occupational safety and health obvious? Perhaps by understanding factors that lead to diverse perceptions, we can become more tolerant of individuals who do not appear to share our opinion or viewpoint. Perhaps the person factors discussed here increase your appreciation and respect for diversity,

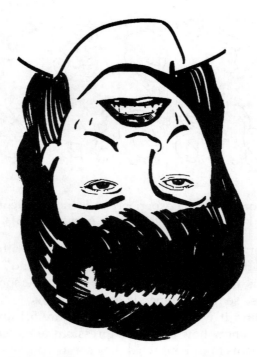

Figure 5.5 Viewing this face from a different orientation (by turning the book
              upside down) will influence a different perception.

and support the basic need to actively listen. "Seek first to understand, before being
understood" is Covey's fifth habit for highly effective people (Covey, 1989, p. 235).

It's also possible that this discussion and the exercises on personal perception
have reduced your tendency to blame individuals for an injury or to look for a single
root cause of an undesirable incident. Before we react to an incident or injury with
our own viewpoint, recommendation, or corrective action, we need to ask others
about their perceptions.

I hope I have not reduced your optimism toward achieving a Total Safety Culture.
Maybe I have alerted you to challenges not previously considered. If I have not
convinced you yet to stop claiming "All injuries are preventable," the next section
should do the trick.

Perceived risk

People are generally underwhelmed or unimpressed by risks or safety hazards at
work. Why? Our experiences on the job lead us to perceive a relatively low level of
risk. This is strange. After all, it is quite probable someone will eventually be hurt on
the job when you factor in the number of hours workers are exposed to various
hazards.

In Chapter 4, I discussed one major reason for low perceptions of risk in the
workplace. It's elemental, really — we usually get away with risky behavior. As
each day goes by without receiving an injury, or even a near hit, we become

more accepting of the common belief "It's not going to happen to me." Now, let's further explore why we are generally not impressed by safety hazards at work.

Real vs. perceived risk

Estimating the risk of injury from working with certain equipment is difficult to determine, because work situations vary so dramatically. Plus, the risk can be eliminated completely by the use of appropriate protective clothing or equipment. Still, many people do not appreciate the value of using PPE or following safe operating procedures. Their perception of risk is generally much lower than actual risk. This thinking pervades society.

Automobile crashes are the nation's leading cause of lost productivity, greater than AIDS, cancer, and heart disease. But, how many of us take driving for granted? The risk of a fatality from driving a vehicle or working in a factory is much higher than from the environmental contamination of radiation, asbestos, or industrial chemicals. Yet, look at the protests over asbestos in schools and neighborhood chemical plants.

Researchers of risk communication have found that various characteristics of a hazard, irrelevant to actual risk, influence people's perceptions. It's important to consider these characteristics because behavior is determined by perceived rather than actual risk.

Figure 5.6 shows factors that influence our risk perceptions. It's derived from research by Drs. Peter Sandman (1991) and Paul Slovic (1991) and their colleagues. The factors listed on the left reduce perceptions of risk and are typically associated with the workplace. The opposing factors in the right-hand column have been found to increase risk perception and are not usually experienced in the work setting. As a consequence, our perception of risk on the job is not as high as it should be, and therefore, we do not work as defensively as we should. Discussing some of these factors will reveal strategies for increasing our own and others' perceptions of risk in certain situations.

The power of choice

Hazards we choose to experience (like driving, skiing, and working) are seen as less risky than ones we feel forced to endure (like food preservatives, environmental pollution, and earthquakes). Of course, the perception of choice is also subjective, varying dramatically among individuals. For example, people who feel they have the freedom to pull up stakes and move whenever they want would likely perceive less risk from a nearby nuclear plant or seismic fault. Likewise, employees who feel they have their pick of places to work generally perceive less risk in a work environment. They are typically more motivated and less distressed. In the next chapter, I discuss relationships among perceived choice, stress, and distress.

Familiarity breeds complacency

Familiarity is probably a more powerful determinant of perceived risk than choice. The more we know about a risk, the less it threatens us. Remember how attentive you were when first learning to drive, or when you were first introduced to the equipment in your workplace? It was not long before you lowered your perceptions of risk, and

Lower Risk	Higher Risk
• exposure is voluntary	• exposure is mandatory
• hazard is familiar	• hazard is unusual
• hazard is forgettable	• hazard is memorable
• hazard is cumulative	• hazard is catastrophic
• collective statistics	• individual statistics
• hazard is understood	• hazard is unknown
• hazard is controllable	• hazard is uncontrollable
• hazard affects anyone	• hazard affects vulnerable people
• preventable	• only reducible
• consequential	• inconsequential

Figure 5.6 Factors on the left reduce perception and are generally associated with the workplace. Adapted from Sandman (1991).

changed your behavior accordingly. When driving, for example, most of us quickly shifted from two hands on the wheel and no distractions to steering with one hand while turning up the radio and carrying on a conversation, even on a cell-phone

The power of publicity

It's so easy to tune out the familiar hazards of the workplace. Safety professionals respond by constantly reminding employees of risks with a steady stream of memos, newsletters, safety meetings, and signs. Still, these efforts cannot compete with the impact of unusual, catastrophic, and memorable events broadcast by the media and dramatized on television and in the movies. Publicity of memorable injuries, like those suffered by John Wayne Bobbitt and Nancy Kerrigan in 1994, influences misperception of actual risk.

Sympathy for victims

Many people feel sympathy for victims of a publicized incident, even vividly visualizing the injury as if it happened to them. Personalizing these experiences increases perceived risk. At work, employees show much more attention and concern for hazards when injuries or near hits are discussed by the coworkers who experienced them, compared to a presentation of statistics. The average person cannot relate to group numbers, but there is power in personal stories. I have met many people over the years who accepted individual accounts in lieu of convincing statistics — "The police officer told Uncle Jake he would have been killed if he had been buckled up"; "Aunt Martha is 91 years old and still smokes two packs of cigarettes a day."

This suggests that we should shift the focus of safety meetings away from statistics, emphasizing instead the human element of safety. Safety talks and intervention strategies should center on individual experiences rather than numbers. This might be easier said than done. Encouraging victims to come forward with their stories is often stifled by management systems in many companies that seem to value fault finding over fact finding, piecemeal rather than system approaches to injury investigation, and enforcement more than recognition to influence on-the-job behaviors.

Understood and controllable hazards

Hazards we can explain and control cause much less alarm than hazards that are not understood and, thus, perceived as uncontrollable. This points up a problem with many employee safety education and training programs. Workplace hazards are explained in a way that creates the impression they can be controlled. Indeed, safety professionals often state a goal of "zero injuries," implying complete control over the factors that cause injuries. This can actually lower perceived risk by convincing people the causes of occupational injuries are understood and controllable.

Perhaps it would be better for safety leaders to admit and publicize that only two of the three types of factors contributing to workplace injuries can be managed effectively — environmental/equipment factors and work behaviors. As I have already discussed in preceding chapters, the mysterious inside, unobservable, and subjective world of people dramatically influences the risk of personal injury. These attitudes, expectancies, perceptions, and personality characteristics cannot be measured, managed, or controlled reliably. Internal human factors make it impossible to prevent all injuries. By discussing the complexity of people and their integral contribution to most workplace hazards and injuries, you can increase both the perceived value of ongoing safety interventions and the belief that a Total Safety Culture requires total commitment and involvement of all concerned.

Acceptable consequences

We are less likely to feel threatened by risk taking or a risk exposure that has its own rewards. But if there are few benefits from an at-risk behavior or environmental condition, outrage — or heightened perceived risk — is likely to be the reaction, along with a concerted effort to prevent or curtail the risk.

Some people, for example, perceive guns, cigarettes, and alcohol as having limited benefit and thus lobby to restrict or eliminate these societal hazards. The availability of and exposure to these hazards will continue, though, as long as a significant number of individuals perceive the risk benefits to outweigh the risk costs. Cost–benefit analyses are subjective and vary widely as a function of individual experience. For example, the two women in Figure 5.7 obviously perceive the consequences of smoking very differently.

On the other hand, the benefits of risky work behaviors are generally obvious to everyone. For example, it's cooler and more comfortable to work without a respirator. It's also convenient and enables a worker to be more productive. The

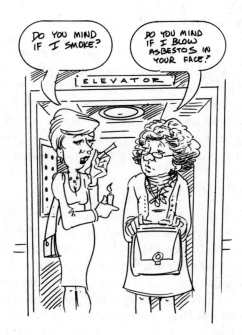

Figure 5.7 The perceived consequences of at-risk behavior can vary widely
from one person to another.

costs of not wearing the mask might be abstract and delayed (if the exposure is not immediately life threatening). Statistics might point out a chance of getting a lung disease, which will not surface for decades, if ever. Decisions about risk taking are made every day by workers. By playing the odds and shooting for short-term gains, risky work practices are often accepted and not perceived to be as dangerous as they really are.

Sense of fairness

Most people believe in a just and fair world. "What goes around comes around." "There's a reason for everything." "People generally get what they deserve." When people receive benefits like increased productivity from their risky behavior, the outrage, public attention, or perceived risk is relatively low. On the other hand, when hazards or injuries seem unfair, as when a child is molested or inflicted with a deadly disease, special attention is given. This increased attention results in more perceived risk.

This makes it relatively easy to obtain contributions or voluntary assistance for programs that target vulnerable populations, like learning-disabled children. The victims of workplace injuries, however, are not perceived as weak and defenseless. Occupational injuries are indiscriminately distributed among employees who take risks, and these people deserve what they get. This is a common perception or attitude and it lowers the outrage we feel when someone gets injured on the job. Lower outrage translates into lower perceived risk.

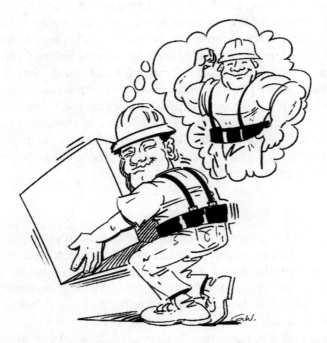

Figure 5.8   Back belts can give a false sense of security.

Risk compensation

A discussion of risk perception would not be complete without examining one of the most controversial concepts in the field of safety. In recent years, it has been given different labels, including *risk homeostasis, risk* or *danger compensation, risk-offsetting behavior,* and *perverse compensation.* Whatever the name, the basic idea is quite simple and straightforward. People are presumed to adjust their behavior to compensate for changes in perceived risk. If a job is made safer with machine guards or the use of PPE, workers might reduce their perception of risk and, thus, perform more recklessly. Figure 5.8 illustrates what I'm talking about in a rather common workplace situation. If the use of a back belt leads to employees lifting heavier loads, then the potential protection from this device could be offset by greater risk taking. The protective device could give a false sense of security and reduce one's perception of being vulnerable to back injury. The result could be more frequent and heavier lifting, and greater probability of injury. This is why the suppliers of back belts emphasize the need for training and education in their proper use.

Implications of risk compensation

I'm convinced from personal experience and reading the research literature that risk compensation is a real phenomenon. What does this mean for injury prevention? Professor Wilde (1994) says it means safety excellence cannot be achieved through top-down rules and enforcement. Some people only follow the rules when they are supervised and might take greater risks when they can get away with it. As the title of his book, *Target Risk,* indicates, Dr. Wilde advocates that safety interventions need to lower the level of risk people are willing to tolerate. This requires a change in values.

Dr. Wilde's position is consistent with the theme of this text. When people understand and accept the paradigm shifts needed for a Total Safety Culture (see Chapter 3), they are on track to reducing their tolerance for risk. Next, they need to believe in the vision of a Total Safety Culture and buy into the mission of achieving it. Then, they need to understand and accept the procedures that can achieve this vision. These methods are explained in Part 3 of this text. Through a continuous process of applying the right procedures, the work force will feel empowered to actively care for a Total Safety Culture. Finally, they will come to treat safety as a value rather than a priority. I discuss these concepts more fully in Part 4.

In conclusion

This chapter explored the concept of selective sensation or perception, and related it to perceived risk and injury control. Visual exercises illustrated the impact of past experience and contextual cues on present perception. This allows us to appreciate diversity and realize the value of actively listening during personal interaction. We need to work diligently to understand the perceptions of others before we impulsively jump to conclusions or attempt to exert our influence.

It's important to realize, however, that people often hold on stubbornly to a preconceived notion about someone or something. As illustrated in Figure 5.9, this bias is often caused by prior experience, and it can dramatically affect perception. Perhaps you know this phenomenon as prejudice, one-sidedness, history, discrimination, pigheadedness, or just plain bias. I like the label "premature cognitive commitment."

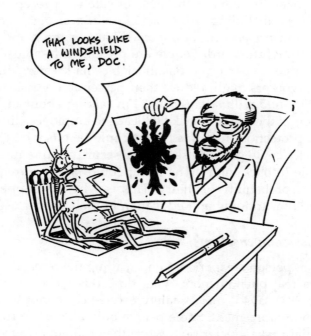

Figure 5.9 We all have premature cognitive commitment.

I like this term because it makes me mindful of the various ingredients of inflexible prejudice. First, it's premature, meaning it is accomplished before adequate diagnosis, analysis, and consideration. Second, it's cognitive, meaning it is a mental process that influences our perceptions, our attitudes, and our behaviors. Finally, it's a commitment. It's not just a fleeting notion or temporary opinion. It's a solid, relatively permanent position or sentiment that affects what information a person seeks, attends to, understands, appreciates, believes, and uses.

Premature cognitive commitment is the root cause of much, if not most, interpersonal conflict. And it's a barrier we must overcome to develop the interdependent teamwork needed to achieve a Total Safety Culture. Being mindful of premature cognitive commitment in ourselves and others will not stop this bias, but it's a start.

We must realize that perceptions of risk vary dramatically among individuals. And we cannot improve safety unless people increase their perception of, and reduce their tolerance for, risk. Changes in risk perception and acceptance will occur when individuals get involved in achieving a Total Safety Culture with the principles and procedures discussed in this book.

Several factors were discussed in this chapter that affect whether employees react to workplace hazards with alarm, apathy, or something in between. Taken together, these factors shape personal perceptions of risk and illustrate why the job of improving safety is so daunting. This justifies more resources for safety and health programs, as well as intervention plans to motivate continual employee involvement. I discuss various intervention approaches in Part 4. But before discussing strategies to fix the problem, we need to understand how stress, distress, and personal attributions contribute to the problem. That's our topic for the next chapter.

chapter six

Stress vs. distress

Stressors can contribute to a near hit or an injury; they are barriers to achieving a Total Safety Culture. However, stressors can provoke positive stress rather than negative distress, which can lead to constructive problem solving rather than destructive, at-risk behavior. This chapter explains the important distinction between stress and distress, and defines factors which determine the occurrence of one or the other.

The concept of "attribution" is introduced as a cognitive process we use to turn stressors into positive stress or negative distress. Attribution bias can reduce distress, but it can also prevent a constructive analysis of an injury or property damage incident. This chapter explains the benefits and liabilities of such bias and shows its role in shifting stress to distress or vice versa.

> "Even if you're on the right track,
> you'll get run over if you just sit there." — Will Rogers

Judy was tired and worried. She had just left her six-year-old son at her sister's house with instructions for her to take him to Dr. Slayton's office for a 10:30 a.m. appointment. She had been up much of the night with Robbie, attempting to comfort him. With tears in his eyes, he had complained of a "hurt" in his stomach. This was the third night his cough had periodically awakened her, but last night Robbie's cough was deeper, seemingly coming from his lungs.

Judy arrived at her workstation a little later than normal and found it more messy than usual. Grumbling under her breath that the night shift had been "careless, sloppy, and thoughtless," she downed her usual cup of coffee and waited for the production line to crank up. She did not clean the work area. After all, it was not her mess. The graveyard shift is not nearly as busy as the day shift. How could they be so sloppy and inconsiderate?

Judy was ready to start her inspection and sorting when she noticed the "load cart" was misaligned. She inserted a wooden handle in the bracket and pulled hard to jerk the cart in place. Suddenly the handle broke, and Judy fell backward against the control panel. Fortunately, she was not hurt, and the only damage was the broken handle. Judy discarded it, inserted another one, and put the cart in place.

During lunch Judy called the doctor's office and learned that her son had the flu, and would be fine in a day or two. She completed the day in a much better mood, without incident.

At the end of her shift, Judy filled out a near-hit report on her morning mishap. She wrote that someone on the graveyard shift had left her work area in disarray, including a misaligned load tray. She also indicated that the design of the cart handle made damage likely; in the past other cart handles had been broken. She recommended a redesign of the handle brackets and immediate discipline for the graveyard shift in her work area.

The fact that Judy filled out a near-hit report is certainly good news, but was this a complete report? Were there some personal factors within Judy that could have influenced the incident? Was Judy under stress or distress and, if so, could this have been a contributing factor? Actually, it has been estimated that from 75 to 85 percent of all industrial injuries can be partially attributed to inappropriate reactions to stress. Furthermore, stress-related headaches are the leading cause of lost-work time in the United States.

Judy's near-hit report was also clearly biased by common attribution errors researched by social psychologists and used by all of us at some time to deflect potential criticism and reduce distress. Attribution errors, along with stress and distress, represent potential barriers to achieving a Total Safety Culture.

What is stress?

In simple terms, stress is a psychological and physiological reaction to events or situations in our environment. Whatever triggers the reaction is called a *stressor*. So stress is the reaction of our minds and bodies to stressors such as demands, threats, conflicts, frustrations, overloads, or changes.

Figure 6.1 depicts a scene that might seem familiar — perhaps too familiar. So many people with so much to do and not enough time to do it. Then our goals are thwarted, and our stress turns to distress. Such frustration can lead to aggression and a demeanor that only increases our distress. It's a vicious cycle, and it certainly increases our propensity for personal injury. Certain personality characteristics referred to as "Type A" are more likely to experience the time urgency and competitiveness depicted in Figure 6.1, and these are associated with higher risk for coronary disease.

Constructive or destructive?

We usually talk about stress in negative terms, something unwanted and uncomfortable. But the first definition of stress in my copy of *The American Heritage Dictionary* (1991) is "importance, significance, or emphasis placed on something" (page 1205). Similarly, *The New Merriam-Webster Dictionary* (1989) defines stress as "a factor that induces bodily or mental tension ... a state induced by such a stress ... urgency, emphasis" (page 701).

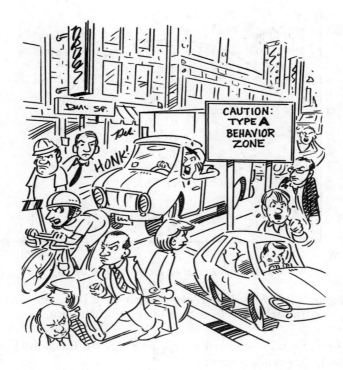

Figure 6.1 Certain environmental conditions and personality
states contribute to stress and distress.

The bad state is distress. Distress is defined as "anxiety or suffering . . . severe strain resulting from exhaustion or an accident" (*The American Heritage Dictionary*, 1991, page 410) or "suffering of body or mind: pain, anguish: trouble, misfortune . . . a condition of desperate need" (*The New Merriam-Webster Dictionary*, 1989, page 224).

Psychological research supports these distinctions between stress and distress. Stress can be positive, giving us heightened awareness, sharpened mental alertness, and an increased readiness to perform. Certain psychological theories presume that some stress is necessary for people to perform. The person who asserts, "I work best under pressure," understands the motivational power of stress. But can too much pressure, too many deadlines, be destructive?

I am sure most of you have been in situations — or predicaments — where the pressure to perform seemed overwhelming. This is the point where too much pressure can hurt performance, where stress becomes distress. The relationship between external stimulation or pressure to perform and actual performance is depicted in Figure 6.2. This inverted U-shaped function is known as the Yerkes-Dodson Law (Yerkes and Dodson, 1908).

The Yerkes-Dodson law states that, up to a point, performance will increase as arousal, or pressure to perform well, increases, but the best performance comes when arousal is optimum rather than maximum. Push a person too far and his performance starts to deteriorate. In fact, at exceptionally high levels of pressure or tension a person might perform as poorly as when he is hardly stimulated at all. Ask someone who is

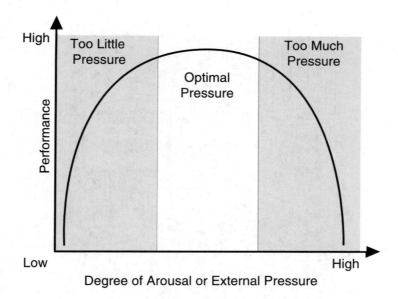

Figure 6.2 Arousal from external pressure (or a stressor)
improves performance to an optimal point.

hysterical and someone who is about to fall asleep to do the same job, and you will
not be pleased by either one's results.

Hans Selye, the Austrian-born founder of stress research said, "Complete freedom
from stress is death" (Selye, 1974). It is extreme, disorganizing stress we need to avoid.
Watch out for distress.

The eye of the beholder

Perceptions play an important role in stress and distress. The boss gives a group of
employees a deadline; some tighten up inside, others take it in stride. Some circle
their calendars and cannot take their minds off the due date. Others seem to pay it
no mind.

When a stressor is noticed and causes a reaction, the result can be constructive or
destructive. If we believe we are *in control* — that we can deal with the overload,
frustrations, conflicts, or whatever is triggered by the stressor — we become
aroused and motivated to go beyond the call of duty. We actually achieve more.
On the other hand, when we believe we cannot handle the demands of the stressor,
the resulting psychological and physiological reactions are likely to be detrimental to
our performance and our health and safety.

Why does a manager's deadline motivate one person and distress another? It
depends on a number of internal person factors. These include the amount of arousal
already present in the individual and the person's degree of preparedness or self-
confidence.

Those "butterflies" we feel in our stomach can help or hinder performance,
depending on personal perception. When the "butterflies" are aligned for goal-
directed behavior, we feel in control of the situation: prepared for it or challenged by

it. The stress is positive — it arouses or motivates performance improvement. When the "butterflies" are misaligned and scattered in different directions, we feel unprepared, burdened rather than challenged. Stress is experienced as distress. This arousal can divert our attention, interfere with thinking processes, disrupt performance, and reduce our ability and overall motivation to perform well. The result can be at-risk behavior and a serious injury.

Identifying stressors

Stress or distress can be provoked by a wide range of demands and circumstances. Some stressors are acute sudden life events, such as death or injury to a loved one, marriage, marital separation or divorce, birth of a baby, failure in school or at work, or a job promotion or relocation. Other stressors include the all-too-frequent minor hassles of everyday life, from long lines and excessive traffic (Figure 6.1) to downsized work conditions and worries about personal finances.

Our jobs or careers are filled with stressors. Consider for a moment how much time you spend working or thinking about your work. Some workplace stressors are obvious; others might not be as evident but are just as powerful. Work overload can obviously become a stressor and provoke either stress or distress, but what about "work underload"? Being asked to do too little can produce profound feelings of boredom, which can also lead to distress. Performance appraisals are stressors that can be motivational if perceived as objective and fair, or they can contribute to distress and inferior performance if viewed as subjective and unfair.

Other work-related factors that can be perceived as stressors and lead to distress and eventual burnout include role conflict or ambiguity; uncertainty about one's job responsibilities; responsibility for others; a crowded, noisy, smelly, or dirty work environment; lack of involvement or participation in decision making; interpersonal conflict with other employees; and insufficient support from coworkers.

Let's review the key points about stress and distress. Actually, the flow schematic in Figure 6.3 says it all. First an environmental event is perceived and appraised as a stressor to be concerned about or as a harmless or irrelevant stimulus. An event is perceived as a stressor if it involves *harm* or loss that has already occurred, a *threat* of some future danger, or a *challenge* to be overcome.

Harm is how we appraise the impact of an event. For example, if you oversleep and miss an important safety meeting, the damage is done. In contrast, *threat* is how we assess potential future harm from the event. Missing the safety meeting could lower your team's opinion of you and reduce your opportunity to get actively involved in a new safety process. *Challenge* is our appraisal of how well we can eventually profit from the damage done. You could view missing the safety meeting as an opportunity to learn from one-on-one discussions with coworkers. This could demonstrate your personal commitment to the safety process and allow you to collect diverse opinions.

In this case, you are perceiving the stressor as an opportunity to learn and show commitment. This evaluation occurs during the secondary appraisal stage and the result can be positive and constructive. On the other hand, your appraisal could be downbeat — you see no recourse for missing the safety meeting, and so you do nothing about it. Now, coworkers might think you do not care about the new safety process

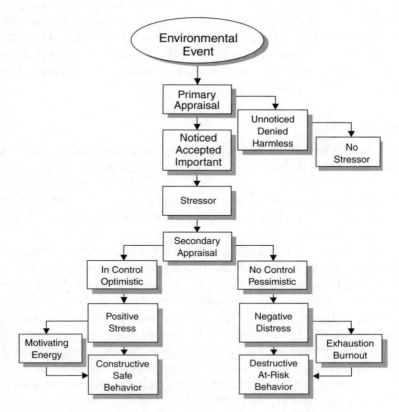

Figure 6.3 Through personal appraisal, people transform stressors into positive stress or negative distress.

and withdraw their support. In turn, you might give up or actively resist participating. This outcome would be nonproductive, of course, and possibly destructive.

The secondary appraisal stage, as depicted in Figure 6.3, determines whether the stressor leads to positive stress and constructive behavior or to negative stress and destructive behavior. The difference rests with the individual. Does he or she assess the stressful situation as controllable and, thus, remains optimistic during attempts to cope with the stressor? As illustrated in Figure 6.4, when people judge their stressors as uncontrollable and unmanageable, a helpless or pessimistic attitude can prevail and lead to distress and destructive or even at-risk behavior. Several personal, interpersonal and environmental factors influence whether this secondary appraisal leads to constructive or destructive behavior. This is the theme of the next section.

Coping with stressors

Understanding the multiple causes of conflict, frustration, overload, boredom, and other potential stressors in our lives can sometimes lead to effective coping mechanisms. These include:

- Revising schedules to avoid hassles like traffic and shopping lines
- Refusing a request that will overload us

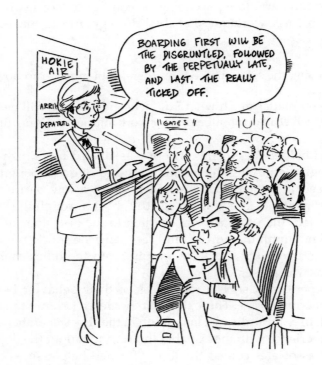

Figure 6.4 Lack of perceived control can lead to distress.

- Finding time to truly relax and recuperate from tension and fatigue
- Communicating effectively with others to clarify work duties, reduce conflict, gain support, or feel more comfortable about added job duties
- Getting reassigned to a task that better fits our present talents and aspirations

The fact is, though, it's often impossible to avoid sudden (acute) or continual (chronic) stressors in our lives. We need to deal with these head-on. Believing you can handle the harm, threat, or challenge of stressors is the first step toward experiencing stress rather than distress, and acting constructively rather than destructively.

Person factors

Certain personality characteristics make some people more resistant to distress. Individuals who believe they control their own destinies and generally expect the best from life are, in fact, more likely to gain control of their stressors and experience positive stress rather than distress. It's important to realize that these person factors — self-mastery and optimism — are not permanent inborn traits of people. They are states of mind or expectations derived from personal experience, and they can be nurtured. It's possible to give people experiences that increase feelings of being "in control" — experiences that lead people to believe something good will come from their attempts to turn stress into constructive action.

Learning to feel helpless. When I help clients assess the safety climate of their workplaces, I often uncover an attitude among hourly workers, and some managers as well, that reflects an important psychological concept called "learned helplessness." For instance, when I ask workers what they do regularly to make their workplace safer, I often hear:

> "Besides following the safety procedures there's not much I can do for safety around here."
> "It really doesn't matter much what I do, whatever will be will be."
> "There's not much I can do about reducing work injuries; if it's my time, it's my time."

This is learned helplessness. The concept was labeled more than 20 years ago by research psychologists studying the learning process of dogs (Seligman, 1975). They measured the speed at which dogs learned to jump a low barrier separating two chambers in order to avoid receiving an electric shock through the grid floor. A tone or light was activated, then a shock was applied to the grid floor of the chamber. At first, the dogs did not jump the hurdle until receiving the shock, but after a few trials the dogs learned to avoid the shock by jumping into the other chamber as soon as the warning signal was presented.

Some dogs experienced shocks regardless of their behavior before the regular shock-avoidance learning trials. These dogs did not learn to jump the barrier to escape the shock. Instead, they typically just laid down in the shock chamber and whimpered. The earlier bad experience with inescapable shocks had taught the dogs to be helpless. Dr. Seligman and associates coined the term "learned helplessness" to describe this state. Their finding has been demonstrated in a variety of human experiments as well.

Note how prior failures conditioned experimental subjects ranging from dogs to humans to feel helpless, in fact, to *be* helpless. It's rather easy to assume that workers develop a "helpless" perspective regarding safety as a result of bad past experiences. If safety suggestions are ignored, or policies and procedures always come from management, workers might learn to feel helpless about safety. It's also true, however, that life experiences beyond the workplace can shape an attitude of learned helplessness. Certain individuals will come to work with a greater propensity to feel helpless in general, and this can carry over to feelings regarding occupational safety and health.

Learned optimism. A bad experience does not necessarily lead to an attitude of learned helplessness. You probably know people who seem to derive strength or energy from their failures, and try even harder to succeed when given another chance. Similarly, Seligman and colleagues found that certain dogs resisted learned helplessness if they previously had success avoiding the electric shock. So it is that some people tend to give up in the face of a stressor, while others fight back.

You probably recognize this difference between learned helplessness and learned optimism as the more popular pessimist vs. optimist distinction. As you have heard it asked before, "How do you see the glass of water?" Is it half full or half empty? We see it differently, depending on our current state of optimism or pessimism. This contrast in personal perception is illustrated humorously in Figure 6.5. The point is that our personality, past experience, and current situation influence whether we feel optimistic and in control or pessimistic and out of control.

What can be done to help those who feel helpless? How can we get them to commit to and participate in the proactive processes of injury prevention? The work

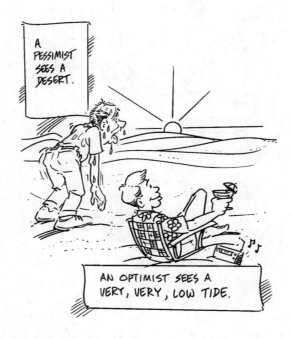

Figure 6.5 Perception affects expectation, which affects behavior, which,
in turn, affects perception.

climate can play a critical role here. This happens when employees are empowered
to make a difference and perceive they are successful.

When workers believe through personal experience their efforts can make a difference in safety, they develop an antidote for learned helplessness. This has been
termed "learned optimism." If the corporate climate empowers workers to take control
and manage safety for themselves and their coworkers, they can legitimately attribute
safety success to their own actions. This bolsters learned optimism and feelings of
being in control. Besides seeing the glass as half full, optimistic people under stress
find ways to fill the rest of the glass.

Fit for stressors

Fitness is another way to increase our sense of personal control and optimism. Being
physically fit increases our body's ability to cope with the fight-or-flight syndrome
discussed earlier. You probably know the basic guidelines for improving fitness,
which include stop smoking; reduce or eliminate alcohol consumption; exercise regularly, at least 3 times a week for about 30 minutes per session; eat balanced meals
with decreased fat, salt, and sugar; do not skip breakfast; and obtain enough sleep
(usually 7 or 8 hours per 24-hour period for most people). Some of us find that

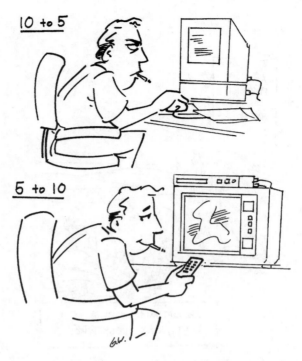

Figure 6.6 Becoming a "mouse potato" by day and a "couch potato" by night can reduce one's physical ability to cope with stressors.

following these guidelines over the long haul is easier said than done. We need support and encouragement to break a smoking or drinking habit or to maintain a regular exercise routine.

Figure 6.6 illustrates the type of behavior that has come with the computer revolution. Low physical activity has become the way of work life for many of us. Often this inactivity spills over into home life. Survey research has shown that only one in five Americans exercises regularly and intensely enough to reduce the risk of stressor-induced heart disease. Figure 6.6 also depicts smoking behavior, considered to be the largest preventable cause of illness and premature death (before age 65) in the United States, and accounting for approximately 125,000 deaths each year.

Also portrayed in Figure 6.6 is the positive influence of perceived control. Although the behavior is essentially the same at work (10 to 5) and at home (5 to 10), the individual is seemingly much happier at home. Why? Because at home he holds the remote control and therefore perceives more personal control.

But personal control is truly in the eyes of the beholder. Figure 6.7 depicts legitimate perceptions of control from the subjects of an experiment. These rodents are not usually considered "in control" of the situation but in many ways they are. By simply changing our perspective, we can often perceive and accept more personal control at work and this can turn negative distress into positive stress.

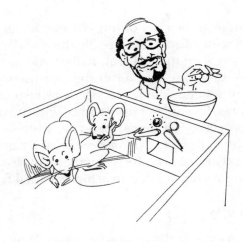

MAN, DO WE HAVE THIS
GUY CONTROLLED, EVERY TIME
WE PULL THE LEVER HE GIVES US
A FOOD PELLET.

Figure 6.7 Even the most obvious top-down situation allows for perceptions
of bottom-up control.

Social factors

A support system of friends, family, and coworkers can do wonders at helping us
reduce distress in our lives. Social support can motivate us to do what it takes to stay
physically fit, and the people around us can make a boring task bearable and even
satisfying. Of course, they can also turn a stimulating job into something dull and
tedious. It works both ways. People can motivate us or trigger conflict, frustration,
hostility, a win–lose perspective, and distress. It's up to us to make the most of the
people around us. We can learn from those who take effective control of stressful
situations and expect the best, or we can listen to the complaining, backstabbing, and
cynicism of others and fuel our own potential for distress.

It's obviously important to interact with those who can help us build resistance
against distress and help us feel better about potential stressors. We can also set the
right example and be the kind of social support to others that we want for ourselves.
The good feelings of personal control and optimism you experience from reaching
out to help others can do wonders in helping you cope with your own stressors. This
actively caring stance builds your own support system, which you might need if your
own stressors get too overwhelming to handle yourself.

The next section of this chapter introduces another means of reducing distress. It
is a phenomenon that has particular implications for safety. In the aftermath of an
injury or near hit, it can distort reports and incident analyses. This results in inappropriate or less than optimal suggestions for corrective action. This phenomenon of
attributional bias can also create communication barriers between people and limit
the cooperative participation needed to achieve a Total Safety Culture.

Attributional bias

Think back to the anecdote at the start of this chapter. I suggested that Judy's near-hit report was incomplete or biased. Specifically, Judy did not report the potential influence of her own distress on the incident. Rather, she focused on factors outside her immediate control — the poor bracket design for the wooden handle and the messy work area left by others. Giving up personal responsibility eliminated the incident as a stressor for her. She did not have to deal with any guilt for almost hurting herself and damaging property. Her denial eased her distress but biased the near-hit report. Psychologists refer to this as an *attributional bias*. By understanding when and how this phenomenon occurs, we can focus injury analysis on finding facts — not faults. This is a paradigm shift needed to achieve a Total Safety Culture.

The fundamental attribution error

Every day, we struggle to explain the actions of others. Why did she say that to me? Why did the job applicant refuse to answer that question? Why did Joe leave his work station in such a mess? Why did the secretary hang up on me? Why did Gayle take sick leave? Why does she allow her young children to ride in the bed of her pick-up truck? Why did the motorist pull a gun out of his glove compartment to shoot someone in the next car? Why were Nicole Brown-Simpson and Ronald Goldman murdered so brutally? In trying to answer questions like these, we point to external environmental factors, such as equipment malfunctioning, excessive traffic, warm climate, and work demands, or to internal person factors, such as personality, intelligence, attitude, or frustration.

Social psychologists have discovered a *fundamental attribution* error when systematically studying how people explain the behavior of others. When evaluating others, we tend to overestimate the influence of internal factors and underestimate external factors. We are more apt to judge the job applicant as rude or unaware (internal factors) than caught off guard by a confusing or unclear question (external factor). Joe was sloppy or inconsiderate rather than overwhelmed by production demands. The injured employee was careless rather than distracted by a sudden environmental noise.

That is how we see things when we are judging others. It's different when we evaluate ourselves. The individuals performing the behaviors in the previous paragraph would say the causes were due more to external than internal factors.

Here's an example. My university students are quick to judge me as being an extrovert — outgoing and sociable. When I lecture in large classes of 600 to 800 students I'm animated and enthusiastic, and they attribute my performance to internal personality traits, but I know better. I see myself in many different situations and realize just how much my behavior changes depending on where I am. In many social settings I'm downright shy and reserved. I'm very sensitive to external influences.

The self-serving bias

Students who flunk my university exams are quick to blame external factors, like tricky questions, wrong reading material assigned, and unfair grading. In contrast, students who do well are quite willing to give themselves most of the credit. It was not that I taught them well or that the exam questions were straightforward and fair;

rather, the student is intelligent, creative, motivated, and prepared. This real-world example, which I bet most readers can relate to, illustrates another type of attributional distortion, referred to as the *self-serving bias.*

How does this bias affect incident or injury analysis? Think of Judy's near-hit experience. She protected her self-esteem by overestimating external causes and underplaying internal factors. People will go to great lengths to shake blame for unintentional property damage or injury. This reduces negative stress or distress. No one wants to feel responsible for a workplace injury, especially if the company puts heavy emphasis on reducing "the numbers," such as the plant's total recordable injury rate.

It's important for us to acknowledge how perceptions can be biased. Outsiders tend to blame the victim; victims look to extenuating circumstances. We should empathize with the self-serving bias of the victim because it will reduce the person's distress. It will shift attention to external factors that can be controlled more easily than internal factors related to a person's attitude, mood, or state of mind.

In conclusion

In this chapter, I explained the difference between stress and distress and discussed some strategies for reducing distress or turning negative distress into positive stress. Stress and distress begin with a stressor which can be a major life event or a minor irritation of everyday living. You can evaluate or appraise the stressor in a way that is constructive, resulting in safe behavior, or destructive, causing at-risk behavior. When people are physically fit, in control, optimistic, and able to rely on the social support of others, they are most likely to turn a stressor into energy for achieving success. This is positive stress.

When stressors are perceived as insurmountable and unavoidable, distress is likely. Without adequate support from others, this condition can lead to physical and mental exhaustion, at-risk behavior, and unintentional injury to oneself or others. We need to become aware of the potential stressors in our lives and in the lives of our coworkers. In addition, we need to develop personal and interpersonal strategies to prevent distress in ourselves and others.

The work culture, including policies, paradigms, and personnel, can have a dramatic impact on whether victims of near hits, injuries, or other adversities experience stress or distress. The fundamental attribution error, where we overestimate personal factors to explain others' behavior ("Judy broke the handle because she was tired, stressed out, and careless."), can provoke distress and pinpoint the very aspects of an incident most difficult to define and control.

A victim's natural tendency to reveal a self-serving bias when discussing an incident — by putting more emphasis on external, situational causes — should be supported by the work culture. This reduces the victim's distress and puts the focus on the observable factors, including behavior, most readily defined and influenced. I detail processes for doing that in Part 3.

part three

Behavior-based psychology

chapter seven

Basic principles

To achieve a Total Safety Culture, we need to integrate behavior-based and person-based psychology and effect large-scale culture changes. The five chapters in Section 3 explain principles and procedures founded on behavioral research which can be applied successfully to change behaviors and attitudes throughout organizations and communities. This chapter describes the primary characteristics of the behavior-based approach to the prevention and treatment of human problems, and shows their special relevance to occupational safety. The three basic ways we learn are reviewed and related to the development of safe vs. at-risk behaviors and attitudes.

> "One can picture a good life by analyzing one's feelings,
> but one can achieve it only by arranging
> environmental contingencies." — B. F. Skinner

Specific safety techniques can be viewed as possible routes to reach a destination, in our case, a Total Safety Culture. A particular route may be irrelevant or need to be modified substantially for a given work culture. The key is to begin with a complete and accurate map. In other words, it's most important to start with an understanding of the basic principles.

If you recall, our overall map or guiding principle is represented by the Safety Triad (Figure 2.3). Its reference points are the three primary determinants of safety performance — environment, person, and behavior factors. To achieve a Total Safety Culture, we need to understand and pay attention to each.

In Part 2, I addressed a number of person-based factors that can contribute to injuries, including cognitions, perceptions, and attributions. The BASIC ID acronym was introduced in Chapter 4 to express the complexity of human dynamics and the special challenges involved in preventing injuries. Behavior was the first dimension discussed, and it is implicated directly or indirectly in each of the other dimensions. Attitudes, sensations, imagery, and cognitions — the thinking, person side of the Safety Triad — are each influenced by behavior. That's what is meant by the phrase, "acting people into changing their thinking." When we change our behaviors, such as adopting a new strategy or paradigm, certain person factors change, too.

The reverse is also true. Changes in attitudes, sensations, imagery, and cognitions can alter behaviors. However, considerable research has shown that it's easier and more cost effective to "act people into changing their thinking" than the reverse, especially in organizations and community settings.

Primacy of behavior

Whether *treating* clinical problems (such as drug abuse, sexual dysfunction, depression, anxiety, pain, hypertension, and child or spouse abuse) or *preventing* any number of health, social, or environmental ills (from developing healthy and safe lifestyles to improving education and protecting the environment), overt behavior is the focus. Treatment or prevention is based on three basic questions:

1. What behaviors need to be increased or decreased to treat or prevent the problem?
2. What environmental conditions, including interpersonal relationships, are currently supporting the undesirable behaviors or inhibiting desirable behaviors?
3. What environmental or social conditions can be changed to decrease undesirable behaviors and increase desirable behaviors?

Thus, behavior change is both the outcome and the means. It's the desired outcome of treatment or prevention and the means to solving the identified problem.

Reducing at-risk behaviors

Heinrich's well-known Law of Safety implicates at-risk behavior as a root cause of most near hits and injuries (Heinrich et al., 1980). Over the past 20 years, various behavior-based research studies have verified this aspect of Heinrich's Law by systematically evaluating the impact of interventions designed to lower employees' at-risk behaviors. Feedback from behavioral observations was a common ingredient in most of the successful intervention processes, whether the feedback was delivered verbally, graphically by tables and charts, or through corrective action.

The behavior-based approach to reducing injuries is depicted in Figure 7.1. At-risk behaviors are presumed to be a major cause of a series of progressively more serious incidents, from a near hit to a fatality. According to Heinrich's Law, there are numerous risky acts for every near hit, and many more near hits than lost-time injuries. This is fortunate news, but let us not forget that timing or luck is usually the only difference between a near hit and a serious injury.

Typically, behavior change techniques are applied to specific targets. It's necessary, of course, that participants know why targeted behaviors are undesirable and have the physical ability to avoid them. Education and engineering interventions are sometimes needed to satisfy the physical and knowledge factors of Figure 7.1. The execution factors represent the motivational aspect of the problem, and usually require the most attention. In other words, people usually know what at-risk behaviors to avoid and have the ability to do so, but their motivation might be lacking or misdirected. Behavior change techniques are used to align individual and group motivation with avoiding the undesired at-risk behavior.

Values and attitudes form the foundation of the pyramid in Figure 7.1. These obviously critical person factors need to support the safety process. Remember our

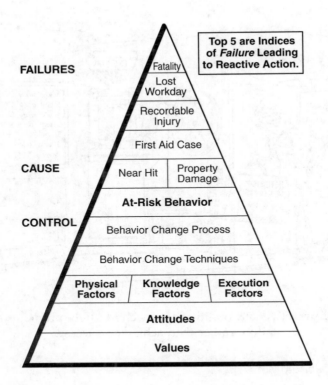

Figure 7.1 Behavior-based safety can decrease at-risk behavior in order to avoid failure.

discussion about risk compensation in Chapter 5 and Wilde's warning that it's more important to reduce risk tolerance than increase compliance with specific safety rules (Wilde, 1994)? This happens when people believe in the safety process and help to make it work. Behavior helps to make the process work and, if involvement is voluntary and appropriately rewarded, it will lead to supportive attitudes and values to keep the process going.

The behavior-based approach illustrated in Figure 7.1 is failure oriented. It's also more reactive than proactive. The outcome measures are failures — fatalities, lost workdays, and the like — that require a fix.

The reactive and punitive approach is typical for government agencies. The most convenient way to control behavior is to pass a law and enforce it. In fact, as depicted in Figure 7.2, this is the standard government approach to safety improvement. When agents of the Occupational Safety and Health Administration (OSHA) visit a site for inspection, they expect to write citations. They look for mistakes or failures, thereby hoping to improve behavior through negative reinforcement. Unfortunately, this perspective can promote negative attitudes about the whole process.

It's usually better to focus on increasing safe behaviors. This is being proactive; when safe behaviors are substituted for at-risk behaviors, injuries will be prevented. By emphasizing safe behaviors, employees feel more positive about the process and are more willing to participate.

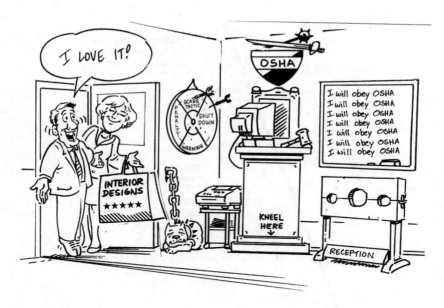

***Figure* 7.2**A reactive and punitive approach to safety promotes avoiding
failure rather than achieving success.

Increasing safe behaviors

Figure 7.3 illustrates a positive and proactive behavior-based model. I do not recommend this instead of the corrective action approach depicted in Figure 7.1. A complete
behavior-based process should target both what is right and wrong about a particular
work routine, but, again, more employees will participate with a positive attitude and
remain committed over time if there is more recognition of achievements than correction of failures.

    Monitoring achievement. The indices of achievement in Figure 7.3 are generally
more difficult to record and track than those in Figure 7.1. Actually, the failure outcomes in Figure 7.1 are observed and recorded quite naturally. Except for near hits
and first-aid cases, the failures in Figure 7.1 have traditionally resulted in systematic
investigation and formal reports. In contrast, the achievements in Figure 7.3 are
somewhat difficult to define and record. In fact, it's impossible to obtain an objective
record of the number of injuries prevented. A reasonable estimate of injuries prevented
can be calculated, though, after you achieve a consistent decrease in injuries as a result
of a proactive, behavior-based process.

    It's possible to derive direct and objective definitions of the other success indices
in Figure 7.3, and to use these to estimate overall achievement. Involvement, for
example, can be defined by recording participation in voluntary programs, and incidents of corrective action can be counted in a number of situations. You can chart the
number of safety work orders turned in and completed, the number of safety audits
conducted and safety suggestions given, and the number of safety improvements
occurring as a result of near-hit reports.

    Safety share. The "safety share" noted in Figure 7.3 is a simple behavior-focused
process that reflects my emphasis on achievement. At the start of group meetings, the

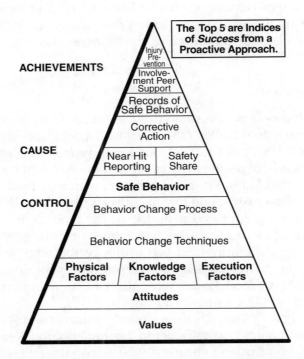

Figure 7.3 Behavior-based safety can increase safe behavior in order to achieve success.

leader asks participants to report something they have done for safety during the past week or since the last meeting. Because the "safety share" is used to open all kinds of meetings, safety is given special status and integrated into the overall business agenda. My experience is that people come to expect queries about their safety accomplishments and many go out of their way to have an impressive safety story to share.

This simple awareness booster — "What have you done for safety?" — helps teach an important lesson. Employees learn that safety is not only loss control (an attempt to avoid failure), but can be discussed in the same terms of achievement as productivity, quality, and profits. As a measurement tool, it's possible to count and monitor the number of safety shares offered per meeting as an estimate of proactive safety success in the work culture.

Learning from experience

A key assumption of the behavior-based approach is that behavior (desirable and undesirable) is learned and can be changed by providing people with new learning experiences. Diverse cultural, social, environmental, and biological factors interact to influence our readiness to learn behaviors. These factors also support or hinder behaviors once they are learned. Although we don't understand exactly how these various factors interact to influence behaviors for each individual, basic ways to develop behavioral patterns have been researched and principles of learning and maintaining human behavior have been formulated.

Psychologists define learning as a change in behavior, or potential to behave in a certain way, resulting from direct and indirect experience. In other words, we learn from observing and experiencing events and behaviors in our environment. While the effects of learning are widespread and varied, it's generally believed there are three basic models: classical conditioning, operant conditioning, and observational learning.

Classical conditioning

This form of learning became the subject of careful study in the early 20th century with the seminal research of Pavlov (1849–1936), a Nobel Prize-winning physiologist from Russia. Pavlov (1927) did not set out to study learning; rather, his research focused on the process of digestion in dogs. He was interested in how reflex responses were influenced by stimulating a dog's digestive system with food. During his experimentation, he serendipitously found that his subjects began to salivate before actually tasting the food. His dogs appeared to anticipate the food stimulation by salivating when they saw the food or heard the researchers preparing it. Some dogs even salivated when seeing the empty food pan or the person who brought in the food. Through experiencing the relationship between certain stimuli and food, the dogs learned when to anticipate food. Pavlov recognized this as an important phenomenum and shifted the focus of his research to address it.

The top half of Figure 7.4 depicts the sequence of stimulus–response events occurring in classical conditioning. Actually, before learning occurs, the sequence includes only three events — conditioned stimulus (CS), unconditioned stimulus (UCS), and unconditioned response (UCR). The UCS elicits a UCR automatically, as in an autonomic reflex. That is, the food (UCS) elicited a salivation reflex (UCR) in Pavlov's dogs. In the same way, the smell of popcorn (UCS) might make your mouth water (UCR), a puff of air to your eye (UCS) would result in an automatic eyeblink (UCR), [ingesting certain drugs (like Antabuse) would elicit a nausea reaction (UCR), and a state trooper writing you a speeding ticket (UCS) is likely to influence an emotional reaction (like distress, nervousness, or anger).*]

If a particular CS consistently precedes the UCS on a number of occasions, the reflex (or involuntary response) will become elicited by the CS. This is classical conditioning and occurred when Pavlov's "slobbering dogs" salivated when they heard the bell that preceded food delivery. Classical conditioning would also occur if your mouth watered (CR) when you heard the bell (CS) from the microwave oven tell you the popcorn was ready, if you blinked your eye (CR) following the illumination of a dim light (CS) that consistently preceded the air puff, if you felt nauseous (CR) after seeing and smelling the alcoholic beverage (CS) that previously accompanied the ingestion of Antabuse, and if you got nervous and upset (CR) after seeing a flashing blue light (CS) in your vehicle's rearview mirror.

Operant conditioning

As shown in the lower portion of Figure 7.4, the flashing blue light on the police car might influence you to press your brake pedal and pull over. This is not an automatic reflex action, but is a voluntary behavior you would perform in order to do what you

---

* The emotional reaction to the police officer is actually learned and really is a CR rather than a UCR. The CR to the blue light (as depicted in Figure 7.4) reflects higher-order conditioning, meaning the police officer acts like a UCR when conditioning the CR to the blue light (the CS).

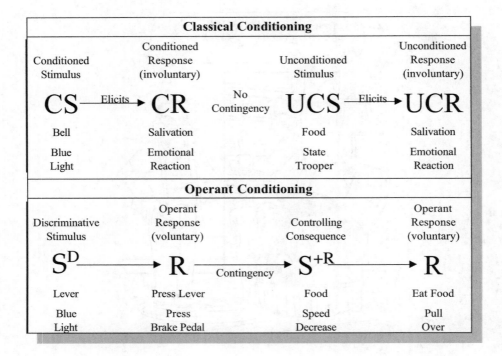

Figure 7.4 The stimulus-response relationships in classical and operant conditioning overlap.

consider appropriate at the time. In other words, you have learned (perhaps indirectly from watching or listening to others or from prior direct experience) to emit certain behaviors when you see a police car with a flashing blue light in your rearview mirror. Of course, you have also learned that certain driving behaviors (like pressing the brake pedal) will give a desired consequence (like slowing down the vehicle), and this will enable another behavior (like pulling over for an anticipated encounter with the police officer).

Selection by consequences. B. F. Skinner (1904–1990), the Harvard professor who pioneered the behavior-based approach to solving societal problems, studied this type of learning by systematically observing the behaviors of rats and pigeons in an experimental chamber referred to as a "Skinner Box" (much to Skinner's dismay). Dr. Skinner termed the learned behaviors in this situation "operants" because they were not involuntary and reflexive, as in classical conditioning, but instead *operated* on the environment to obtain a certain consequence. A key principle demonstrated in the operant learning studies is that voluntary behavior is strengthened (increased) or weakened (decreased) by consequences (events immediately following behaviors).

The relationship between a response and its consequence is a contingency, and this relationship explains our motivation for doing almost everything we choose to do. Thus, the hungry rat in the Skinner Box presses the lever to receive food and the vehicle driver pushes the brake pedal to slow down the vehicle. Indeed, we all select various responses to perform daily — like eating, walking, reading, working, writing, talking, and recreating — to receive the immediate consequences they

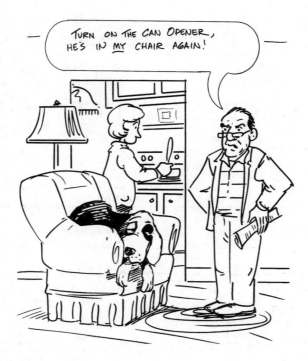

Figure 7.5 Activators direct behavior change when backed up by a consequence.

provide us. Sometimes, we engage in the behavior to achieve a pleasant consequence, such as a reward. Other times, we perform a particular act to avoid an unpleasant consequence — a punisher. We usually stop performing behaviors that are followed by punishers.

The ABC (activator–behavior–consequence) contingency is illustrated in Figure 7.5. The dog will move if he expects to receive food after hearing the sound of the can opener. In other words, the direction provided by an activator is likely to be followed when it is backed by a consequence that is soon, certain, and significant. This is operant conditioning.

Might the dog in Figure 7.5 salivate when hearing the can opener? If the sound of the can opener elicits a salivation reflex in the dog, we have an example of classical conditioning. In this case, the can-opener sound is a CS and the salivation is the CR (*conditioned response*). What is the UCS in this example? Right: The food which previously followed the sound of the electric can opener is the UCS, which elicits the UCR of salivating without any learning experience. This UCS–UCR reflex is natural or "wired in" the organism.

So, an important point illustrated in Figure 7.5 is that operant and classical conditioning often occur simultaneously. While we operate on the environment to achieve a positive consequence or avoid a negative consequence, emotional reactions are often classically conditioned to specific stimulus events in the situation. We learn to like or dislike the environmental context and/or the people involved as a result of the type of ABC contingency influencing ongoing behavior. This is how attitude can be negatively affected by enforcement techniques.

Emotional reactions. As I discussed in Chapter 3, we feel better when working for pleasant consequences than when working to avoid or escape unpleasant consequences. This can be explained by considering the classical conditioned emotions that naturally accompany the agents of reward vs. punishment. How do you feel, for example, when a police officer flashes a blue light to signal you to pull over? When the instructor asks to see you after class? When you enter the emergency area of a hospital? When the dental assistant motions that "you're next"? When your boss leaves you a phone message to "see him immediately"? When you see your family at the airport after returning home from a long trip?

Your reactions to these situations depend, of course, on your past experiences. Police officers, teachers, doctors, dentists, and supervisors do not typically elicit negative emotional reactions in young children. However, through the association of certain cues with the consequences we experience in the situation, a negative emotional response or attitude can develop, and you do not have to experience these relationships directly. In fact, we undoubtedly learn more from observing and listening to others than from first-hand experience. This brings us to the third way in which we learn from experience — observational learning.

Observational learning

A large body of psychological research indicates that this form of learning is involved to some degree in almost everything we do. Whenever you do something a particular way because you saw someone else do it that way, or because someone showed you to do it that way, or because characters on television or in a video game did it that way, you are experiencing observational learning. Whenever you attribute "peer pressure" as the cause of someone taking up an unhealthy habit (like smoking cigarettes or drinking excessive amounts of alcohol) or practicing an at-risk behavior (like driving at excessive speeds or adjusting equipment without locking out the energy source), you are referring to observational learning. When you remind someone to set an example for others, you are alluding to the critical influence of observational learning.

Vicarious consequences. As children, we learned numerous behavioral patterns by watching our parents, teachers, and peers. When we saw our siblings or schoolmates receive rewards like special attention for certain behaviors, we were more likely to copy that behavior, for instance. This process is termed vicarious, or indirect, reinforcement. At the same time, when we observed others getting punished for certain behaviors, we learned to avoid these behaviors. This is referred to as vicarious punishment.

As adults, we teach others by example. As illustrated in Figure 7.6, our children learn new behavior patterns, including verbal behaviors, by watching us and listening to us. In this way they learn what is expected of them in various situations. I have talked with many parents of teenagers who are nervous about their son or daughter getting a driver's license. For some, their concern goes beyond the numerous dangers of real-world driving situations. They realize that several of their own driving behaviors, practiced regularly in front of their children for years, have not been exemplary.

How can we expect our teenagers to practice safe driving and keep their emotions under control if we have shown them the opposite throughout their childhood? Of

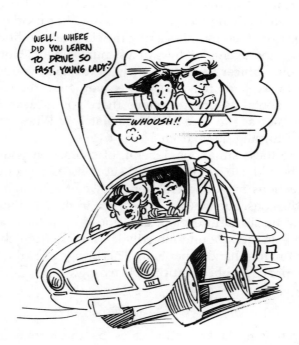

Figure 7.6 Children learn a lot from their parents through observational learning.

course, we are not the only role models who influence our children through observational learning, but we can make a difference.

Our actions influence others to a greater extent than we realize. Without our being aware of our influence, children learn by watching us at home; our coworkers are influenced by our practices at work. Not only does the occurrence of safe acts encourage similar behavior by observers, but verbal behavior can also be influential. If a supervisor is observed commending a worker for her safe behavior or reprimanding an employee for an at-risk practice, observers may increase their performance of similar safety behaviors (through vicarious reinforcement) or decrease the frequency of similar at-risk behavior (through vicarious punishment). Indeed, to make safe behavior the norm — rather than the exception — we must always set an example both in our own work practices and in the verbal consequences we offer coworkers following their safe and at-risk behaviors. Figure 7.7 offers a memorable pictorial regarding the influence of example setting on observational learning.

Overlapping types of learning

Laboratory methodologies have been able to study each type of learning separately, but the real world rarely offers such purity. In life, the usual situation includes simultaneous influence from more than one learning type. The operant learning situation, for example, is likely to include some classical (emotional) conditioning. As I indicated earlier, this is one reason rewarding consequences should be used more frequently than punishing consequences to motivate behavior change.

Remember, a rewarding situation (unconditioned stimulus) can elicit a positive emotional experience (unconditioned response), and a punitive situation (UCS) can

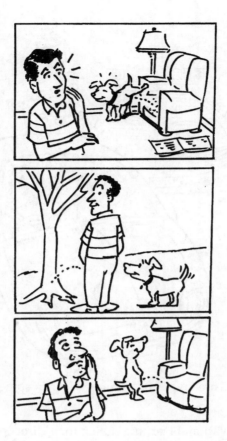

Figure 7.7 Intentionally and unintentionally we teach through our example.

elicit a negative emotional reaction (UCR). With sufficient pairing of rewarding or punishing consequences with environmental cues (such as a work setting or particular people), the environmental setting (conditioned stimulus) can elicit a positive or negative emotional reaction or attitude (conditioned response). This can in turn facilitate (if it is positive) or inhibit (if it is negative) ongoing performance.

Figure 7.8 depicts a situation in which all three learning types occur at the same time. As discussed earlier and diagrammed in Figure 7.4, the blue flashing light of the police car signals drivers to press the brake pedal of their car and pull over. In this case, the blue light is considered a *discriminative stimulus* because it tells people when to respond in order to receive or avoid a consequence. Actually, drivers would apply their brakes to avoid punitive consequences, so this situation illustrates an avoidance contingency where drivers respond to avoid failure.

The flashing blue light might also serve as a conditioned stimulus eliciting a negative emotional reaction. This is an example of classical conditioning occurring simultaneously with operant learning. Our negative emotional reaction to the blue light might have been strengthened by prior observational learning. As a child, we might have seen one of our parents pulled over by a state trooper and subsequently observed a negative emotional reaction from our parent. The children in Figure 7.8 are not showing the same emotional reaction as the driver. Eventually, they will probably

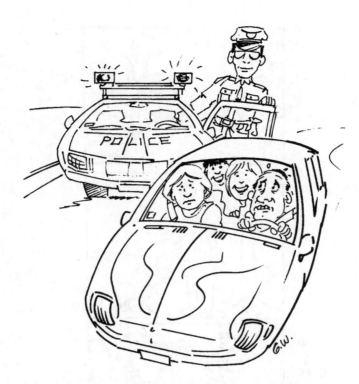

Figure 7.8   Three types of learning occur in some situations.

do so as a result of observational learning. Later, their direct experience as drivers will strengthen this negative emotional response to a flashing blue light on a police car.

In conclusion

In this chapter, I reviewed the basic principles underlying a behavior-based approach to the prevention and treatment of human problems. The behavior-based principles — the primacy of behavior, direct assessment and evaluation, intervention by managers and peers, and three types of learning — were explained with particular reference to reducing personal injury.

Because at-risk behaviors contribute to most if not all injuries, a Total Safety Culture requires a decrease in at-risk behaviors. Organizations have attempted to do this by targeting at-risk acts, exclusive of safe acts, and using corrective feedback, reprimands, or disciplinary action to motivate behavior change. This approach is useful, but less proactive and less apt to be widely accepted than a behavior-based approach that emphasizes recognition of safe behaviors. It will be easier to get employees involved in safety achievement if credit is given for doing the right thing more often than reprimands for doing wrong.

The three types of learning are relevant for understanding safety-related behaviors and attitudes. Most of our safe and at-risk behaviors are learned operant behaviors, performed in particular settings to gain positive consequences or to avoid negative consequences. Classical conditioning often occurs at the same time to link positive or negative emotional reactions with the stimulus cues surrounding the experience of receiving consequences. These cues include the people who deliver the rewards or penalties. We often learn what to do and what not to do by watching others receive recognition or correction for their operant behaviors. This is observational learning, an ongoing process that should motivate us to try to set the safe example at all times.

chapter eight

Identifying critical behaviors

The practical "how to" aspects of this book begin with this chapter. The overall process is called DO IT, each letter representing the four basic components of a behavior-based approach: Define *target behaviors to influence;* Observe *these behaviors;* Intervene *to increase or decrease target behaviors; and* Test *the impact of your intervention process. This chapter focuses on developing a critical behavior checklist for objective observing, intervening, and testing.*

"As I grow older, I pay less attention to what men say, I just watch what they do."
— Andrew Carnegie

Now the action begins. Up to this point, I have been laying the groundwork (rationale and theory) for the intervention strategies described here and in the next three chapters. From this information, you will learn how to develop action plans to increase safe behaviors, decrease at-risk behaviors, and achieve a Total Safety Culture.

Why did it take me so long to get here — to the implementation stage? Indeed, if you are looking for "quick-fix" tools to make a difference in safety you may have skipped or skimmed the first two parts of this text and started your careful reading here. I certainly appreciate that the pressures to get to the bottom line quickly are tremendous but, remember, there is no quick fix for safety. The behavior-based approach that is the heart of this book is the most efficient and effective route to achieving a Total Safety Culture. It is a never ending continuous improvement process, one that requires ongoing and comprehensive involvement from the people protected by the process. In industry, these are the operators or line workers.

Long-term employee participation requires understanding and belief in the principles behind the process. Employees must also perceive that they "own" the procedures that make the process work. For this to happen it is necessary to teach the principles and rationale first (as done in this book), and then work with participants to develop specific process procedures. This creates the perception of ownership and leads to long-term involvement.

When people are educated about the principles and rationale behind a safety process, they can customize specific procedures for their particular work areas. Then the relevance of the training process is obvious and participation is enhanced. People are more likely to accept and follow procedures they helped to develop. They see such safe operating procedures as "the best way to do it" rather than "a policy we must obey because management says so."

As we begin here to define principles and guidelines for action plans, it's important to keep one thing in mind — you need to start with the conviction that there is rarely a generic best way to implement a process involving human interaction. For a behavior-based safety process to succeed in your setting, you will need to work out the procedural details with the people whose involvement is necessary. The process needs to be customized to fit your culture.

The DO IT process

For well over a decade, I have taught applications of the behavior-based approach to industrial safety with the acronym DO IT. The process is continuous and involves the following four steps:

D: Define the critical target behavior(s) to increase or decrease.
O: Observe the target behavior(s) during a preintervention baseline period to set behavior-change goals and, perhaps, to understand natural environmental or social factors influencing the target behavior(s).
I: Intervene to change the target behavior(s) in desired directions.
T: Test the impact of the intervention procedure by continuing to observe and record the target behavior(s) during the intervention program.

From data obtained in the test phase, you can evaluate the impact of your intervention and make an informed decision whether to continue it, implement another strategy, or define another behavior to target for the DO IT process.

To begin, just what are clear and concise definitions of target behaviors? This is the first step in the DO IT process. There is so much to choose from: using equipment safely, lifting correctly, locking out power appropriately, and looking out for the safety of others, to name just a scant few. The outcome of behaviors, such as wearing PPE, working in a clean and organized environment, and using a vehicle safety belt can also be targeted.

If two or more people independently obtain the same frequency recordings when observing the defined behavior or behavioral outcome during the same time period, you have a definition sufficient for an effective DO IT process. Baseline observations of the target behavior should be made and recorded before implementing an intervention program. More details on this aspect of the process are given later in this chapter.

What about the intervention step? This phase of DO IT involves one or more behavior-change techniques, based on the simple ABC model depicted in Figure 8.1. As I discussed in the preceding chapter, activators direct behavior and consequences motivate behavior. For example, a ringing telephone or doorbell activates the need for certain behaviors from residents, but residents answer or do not answer the telephone or door depending on current motives or expectations developed from prior experiences.

Let's talk a little more about consequences. The strongest consequences are soon, certain, and sizeable. In other words, we work diligently for immediate, probable, and large positive reinforcers or rewards, and we work frantically to escape or avoid soon, certain, and sizable negative reinforcers or punishers. This helps explain why safety is a struggle in many workplaces. You see, safe behaviors are usually *not* reinforced

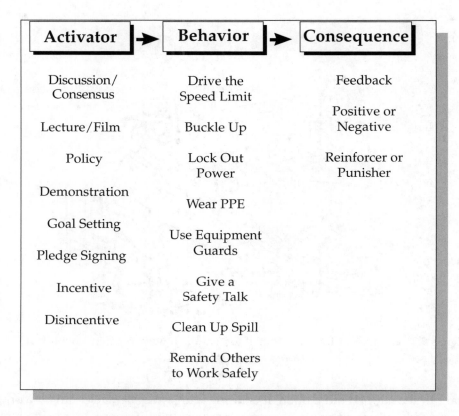

Figure 8.1 The ABC model is used to develop behavior change interventions.

by soon, sizable, and certain consequences. In fact, safe behaviors are often punished by soon and certain *negative* consequences, including inconvenience, discomfort, and slower goal attainment. Also, the consequences that motivate safety professionals to promote safe work practices — reduced injuries and associated costs — are delayed, negative, and uncertain (actually improbable) from an individual perspective.

Check out the two lawn-mower operators in Figure 8.2. Which one is having more fun? Who is more uncomfortable? Who is safe? Chances are both men will complete mowing their lawns without an injury. So which worker will have enjoyed the task more? This defines the fight against human nature discussed earlier in Part 2. Safety typically means more discomfort and inconvenience and less fun than the more efficient at-risk alternative.

The DO IT process is a tool to use in this struggle with human nature. Developing and maintaining safe work practices often requires intervention strategies to keep people safe — strategies involving activators, consequences, or both. But we're getting ahead of ourselves. First, we need to define critical behaviors to establish targets for our intervention. Let's see how this is done.

Defining target behaviors

The DO IT process begins by defining critical behaviors to work on. These become the targets of our intervention strategies. Some target behaviors might be *safe* behaviors

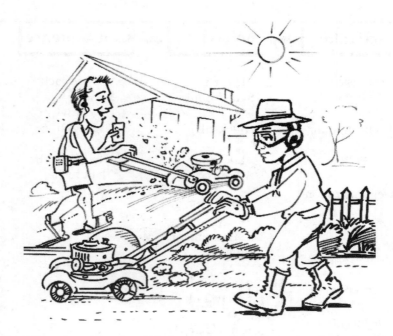

Figure 8.2 Compared to at-risk behavior, safe behavior is often uncomfortable, inconvenient, and less fun.

you want to see happen more often, like lifting with knees bent, cleaning a work area, putting on PPE, or replacing safety guards on machinery. Other target behaviors may be *at-risk* behaviors that need to be decreased in frequency, such as misusing a tool, overriding a safety switch, placing obstacles in an area designated for traffic flow, stacking materials incorrectly, and so on.

A DO IT process can define desirable behaviors to be encouraged or undesirable behaviors to be changed. What the process focuses on in your workplace depends on a review of your safety records, job hazard analyses, near-hit reports, audit findings, interviews with employees, and other useful information.

Deciding which behaviors are critical is the first step of a DO IT process. A great deal can be discovered by examining the workplace and discussing with people how they have been performing their jobs. People already know a lot about the hazards of their work and the safe behaviors needed to avoid injury. They even know which safety policies are sometimes ignored to get the job done on time. They often know when a near hit had occurred because an at-risk behavior or environmental hazard had been overlooked. They also know which at-risk behaviors could lead to a serious injury (or fatality) and which safe behaviors could prevent a serious injury (or fatality).

In addition to employee discussions, injury records and near-hit reports can be consulted to discover critical behaviors (both safe and at risk). Job hazard analyses or standard operating procedures can also provide information relevant to selecting critical behaviors to target in a DO IT process. Obviously, the plant safety director or the person responsible for maintaining records for OSHA or MSHA (Mine Safety and Health Administration) can provide valuable assistance in selecting critical behaviors.

After selecting target behaviors, it's critical to define them in a way that gets everyone on the same page. All participants in the process need to understand exactly what behaviors you intend to support, increase, or decrease. Defining target behaviors results in an objective standard for evaluating an intervention process.

What is behavior?

The key is to define behaviors correctly. Let's begin by stepping back a minute to consider: What is behavior? Behavior refers to acts or *actions* by individuals that can be *observed* by others. In other words, behavior is what a person *does* or *says* as opposed to what he or she thinks, feels, or believes.

Yes, the act of saying words such as "I am tired," is a behavior because it can be observed or heard by others. However, this is not an observation of tired behavior. If the person's work activity slows down or amount of time on the job decreases, we might infer that the person is actually tired. On the other hand, a behavioral "slow down" could result from other internal causes, like worker apathy or lack of interest. The important point here is that feelings, attitudes, or motives should not be confused with behavior. They are *internal* aspects of the person that cannot be directly observed by others. It is risky to infer inner person characteristics from external behaviors.

Describing behaviors

A target behavior needs to be defined in observable terms so multiple observers can independently watch one individual and obtain the same results regarding the occurrence or nonoccurrence of the target behavior. There should be no room for interpretation. "Is not paying attention," "acting careless," or "lifting safely," for example, are not adequate descriptions of behavior because observers would not agree consistently about whether the behavior occurred. In contrast, descriptions like "keeping hand on handrail," "moving knife away from body when cutting," and "using knees while lifting" are objective and specific enough to obtain reliable information from trained observers. In other words, if two observers watched for the occurrence of these behaviors, they would likely agree whether or not the behavior occurred.

Multiple behaviors

Let's look more closely at types of behaviors. Some workplace activities can be treated effectively as a single behavior. Examples include "looking left–right–left before crossing the road," "walking within the yellow safety lines," "honking the fork lift horn at the intersection," "returning tools to their proper location," "bending knees while lifting," and "keeping a hand on the handrail while climbing stairs."

Some outcomes of behaviors also can be dealt with in singular terms, like "using ear plugs," "using a vehicle safety belt," "climbing a ladder that is properly tied off," "working on a scaffold with appropriate fall protection," and "repairing equipment that had been locked out correctly." With a proper definition, an observer could readily count occurrences of these safe behaviors (or outcomes) during a systematic audit.

Many safety activities are made up of more than one discrete behavior, however, and it may be important to treat these behaviors independently in a definition and an audit. "Bending knees while lifting," for example, is only one aspect of a safe lift.

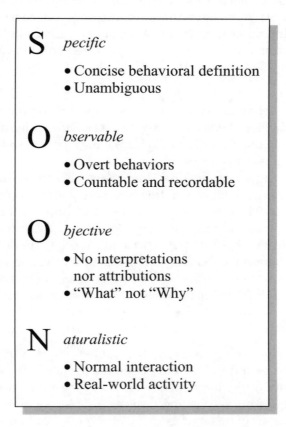

Figure 8.3 Behavioral observations for the DO IT process should be "SOON."

Thus, if safe lifting were the activity targeted in a DO IT process, it would be necessary to define the separate behaviors (or procedural steps) of a safe lift. This would include, at least, checking the load before lifting, asking for help in certain situations, lifting with the legs, holding the load close to one's body, lifting in a smooth motion, and moving feet when rotating (or not twisting).

Each of the procedural steps in safe lifting requires a clear objective definition so two observers could determine reliably whether the behavior in a lifting sequence had occurred. Observing reliably whether the load was held close and knees were bent would be relatively easy. However, defining a "smooth lift" so that observers could agree on 80 percent or more of the observations would be more difficult and, for observers to reliably audit "asking for help," the "certain situations" calling for this response would need to be specified.

Observing behavior

The acronym "SOON" depicted in Figure 8.3 reviews the key aspects of developing adequate definitions of critical behaviors to target for a DO IT process. You are ready for the observation phase when you have a checklist of critical behaviors with definitions that are Specific, Observable, Objective, and Naturalistic. We have already considered most of the characteristics of behavioral definitions implied by these key words, and examples of behavioral checklists are provided later in this chapter, as well as in Chapter 12 on safety coaching.

A personal example

My daughter Krista asked me to drive her to the local Virginia Department of Motor Vehicles office to get her "learner's permit." She was 15 years old and thought she was ready to drive. Of course, I knew better, but how do you fight a culture that puts teenagers behind the wheel of motor vehicles before they are really ready for such a risky situation?

"Don't worry, Dad," my daughter said, "I've had driver's education in high school." Actually, that was part of my worry. She was educated about the concepts and rules regarding driving, but she had not been trained. She had not yet translated her education into operations or action plans.

In order to obtain a license to operate a motor vehicle in Virginia before the age of 18, teenagers with a learner's permit are required to take seven two-hour instructional periods of on-the-road experience with an approved driver-training school. For one-half of these sessions they must be the driver; the rest of the time they sit in the back seat and perhaps learn through observation. Thus, for seven one-hour sessions Krista drove around town with an instructor in the front seat and one or more students in the back, waiting for their turn at the wheel. This was an opportunity for my daughter to transfer her driver education knowledge to actual performance.

Driving activators and consequences. On-the-job training obviously requires an appropriate mix of observation and feedback from an instructor. Practice does *not* make perfect. Only through appropriate feedback can people improve their performance. Some tasks give natural feedback to shape our behavior. When we turn a steering wheel in a particular direction, we see immediately the consequence of our action and our steering behavior is naturally shaped. The same is true of several other behaviors involved in driving a motor vehicle, from turning on lights, windshield wipers, and cruise-control switches to pushing gas and brake pedals.

However, many other aspects of driving are not followed naturally with feedback consequences, particularly those that can prevent injury from vehicle crashes. Although we get feedback to tell us our steering wheel, gas pedal, turn signal lever, and brakes work, we do not get natural feedback regarding our safe vs. at-risk use of such control devices. Therefore, as shown in Figure 8.4, feedback must be added to the driving situation if we want behavior to improve.

Also, when we first learn to drive, we do not readily recognize the activators that should signal the use of various vehicle controls. This is commonly referred to as "judgment." From a behavior-based perspective, "good driving judgment" is recognizing environmental conditions (or activators) that signal certain vehicle-control behaviors, and then implementing the controls appropriately.

I wondered whether my daughter's driving instructor would give her appropriate and systematic feedback regarding her driving "judgment." Would he point out consistently the activators that require safe vehicle-control behaviors? Would he put emphasis on the positive, by supporting my daughter's safe behaviors before criticizing her at-risk behaviors? Would he, or a student in the back seat, display negative

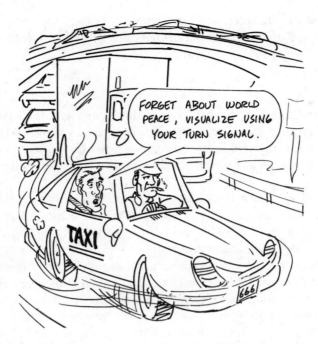

Figure 8.4 Practice requires feedback to make perfect.

emotional reactions in certain situations and teach Krista (through classical condition-ing) to feel anxious or fearful in particular driving situations? Would some at-risk driving behaviors by Krista or the other student drivers be overlooked by the instructor and lead to observational learning that some at-risk driving behaviors are acceptable?

Developing a critical behavior checklist for driving. Even if the driving instruction is optimal, seven hours of such observation and feedback is certainly not sufficient to teach safe driving habits. I recognized a need for additional driving instruction for my daughter. We needed a DO IT process for driving. The first step was to define critical behaviors to target for observation and feedback. Through one-on-one discussion, my daughter and I derived a list of critical driving behaviors and then agreed on specific definitions for each item. My university students practiced using this critical behavior checklist (CBC) a few times with various drivers and refined the list and definitions as a result. The CBC we eventually used is depicted in Figure 8.5.

Using the critical behavior checklist

After refining the CBC and discussing the final behavioral definitions with Krista, I felt ready to implement the second stage of DO IT — observation. I asked my daughter to drive me to the university — about nine miles from home — to pick up some papers. I made it clear I would be using the CBC on both parts of the roundtrip. When we reached the university parking lot, I totaled the safe and at-risk checkmarks and calculated the percentage of safe behaviors. Krista was quite anxious to learn the results and I looked forward to giving her objective behavioral feedback. I had good news. Her percentage of safe driving behaviors (percent safe) was 85 percent and I considered this quite good for our first time.

Critical Behavior Checklist for Driving			
Driver:	Date:		Day:
Observer 1:	Origin:		Start Time:
Observer 2:	Destination:		End Time:
Weather:			
Road Conditions:			
Behavior	**Safe**	**At-Risk**	**Comments**
Safety Belt Use:			
Turn Signal Use:			
Left turn			
Right turn			
Lane change			
Intersection Stop:			
Stop sign			
Red light			
Yellow light			
No activator			
Speed Limits:			
25 mph and under			
25 mph- 35 mph			
35 mph- 45 mph			
45mph- 55 mph			
55mph- 65 mph			
Passing:			
Lane Use:			
Following Distance (2 sec):			
Totals:			

% Safe = $\dfrac{\text{Total Safe Observations}}{\text{Total Safe + At-Risk Obs.}}$ = _____%

Figure 8.5 A critical behavior checklist (CBC) can be used to increase safe driving.

I told Krista her "percent safe" score and proceeded to show her the list of safe checkmarks, while covering the checks in the At-Risk column. Obviously, I wanted to make this a positive experience, and to do this, it was necessary to emphasize the behaviors I saw her do correctly. To my surprise, she did not seem impressed with her 85 percent safe score and pushed me to tell her what she did wrong. "Get to the bottom line, Dad," she asserted, "where did I screw up?" I continued an attempt to make the experience positive, by saying, "You did great, honey; look at the high number of safe behaviors." "But why wasn't my score 100 percent?" reacted Krista. "Where did I go wrong?"

This initial experience with the driving CBC was enlightening in two respects. It illustrated the unfortunate reality that the "bottom line" for many people is "where did I make a mistake?" My daughter, at age 15, had already learned that people evaluating her performance seem to be more interested in mistakes than successes. That obviously makes performance evaluation (or appraisal) an unpleasant experience for many people.

A second important outcome from this initial CBC experience was the realization that people can be unaware of their at-risk behaviors and only through objective feedback can this be changed. My daughter did not readily accept my corrective feedback regarding her four at-risk behaviors. In fact, she vehemently denied that she did not always come to a complete stop. However, she was soon convinced of her error when I showed her my data sheet and my comment regarding the particular intersection where there was no traffic and she made only a rolling stop before turning right. I did remind her that she did use her turn signal at this and every intersection and this was something to be proud of. She was developing an important safety habit, one often neglected by many drivers.

I really did not appreciate the two lessons from this first application of the driving CBC until my daughter monitored my driving. That's right, Krista used the CBC in Figure 8.5 to evaluate my driving on several occasions. I found this reciprocal application of a CBC to be most useful in developing mutual trust and understanding between us. I found myself asking my daughter to explain my lower than perfect score and arguing about one of the recorded at-risk behaviors. I, too, was defensive about being 100 percent safe. After all, I had been driving for 37 years and teaching and researching safety for more than 20 years. How could I not get a perfect driving score when I knew I was being observed?

From our experience with the CBC, my daughter and I learned the true value of an observation and feedback process. While using the checklist does translate education into training through systematic observation and feedback, the real value of the process is the interpersonal coaching that occurs. In other words, we learned not to get too hung up on the actual numbers. After all, there is plenty of room for error in the numerical scores. Rather, we learned to appreciate the fact that through this process people are actively caring for the safety and health of each other in a way that can truly make a difference. We also learned that even experienced people can perform at-risk behavior and not even realize it.

Two basic approaches

The CBC examples described previously illustrate two basic ways of implementing the "define" and "observe" stages of DO IT. The driving CBC I developed with my daughter illustrates the observation and feedback process recommended by a number of successful behavior-based safety consultants. I refer to this approach as one-on-one safety coaching because it involves an observer using a CBC to provide instructive behavioral feedback to another person.

The second approach to the define and observe stages of DO IT involves a limited CBC (perhaps targeting only one behavior) and does not necessarily involve one-on-one coaching. This is the approach used in most of the published studies of the behavior-based approach to safety.

Each of these approaches to the define and observe stages of DO IT is advantageous for different applications within the same culture. Thus, it's important to understand the basic procedures of each and to consider their advantages and disadvantages. For some work settings, I have found it quite useful to start with the simpler approach of targeting only a few CBC behaviors. With immediate success, behaviors are then added until eventually a comprehensive CBC is developed, accepted, and used willingly throughout a worksite.

Starting small

This approach targets a limited number of critical behaviors but does not require one-on-one observation. A work group defines a critical behavior or behavioral outcome to observe, as discussed earlier in this chapter. After defining their target so two or more observers can reliably observe and record a particular property of the behavior

Observer:		Date:	
Target Behavior		Safe	At-Risk
load appropriate			
hold close			
use legs			
move feet - don't twist			
smooth motion - no jerks			
Comments (use back if necessary):			

% Safe Observations:

$$\frac{\text{Total Safe Observations}}{\text{Total Safe Observations} + \text{At-Risk Observations}} \times 100 = \underline{\hspace{2cm}} \%$$

Figure 8.6 A critical behavior checklist (CBC) can be used to increase safe lifting.

(usually frequency of occurrence), the group members should give each other permission to observe this work practice among themselves. If some group members do not give permission, it's best not to argue with them. Simply exclude these individuals from the observations and invite them to join the process whenever they feel ready. They will likely participate eventually when they see that the DO IT process is not a "Gotcha Program" but an objective and effective way to care actively for the safety of others and build a Total Safety Culture.

It helps to develop a behavior checklist to use during observations. As discussed earlier, target behaviors like "safe lifting" and "safe use of stairs" include a few specific behaviors, either safe or at risk. Therefore, the CBC should list each behavior separately and include columns for checking "safe" or "at risk." Figure 8.6 depicts a sample CBC for safe lifting. Through use of this CBC, a work group might revise their definitions and possibly add a lifting-related behavior relevant to their work area.

Participants willing to be observed anonymously for the target behavior(s) use the CBC to maintain daily records of the safe and at-risk behaviors defined by the group. They do not approach another individual specifically to observe him or her. Rather they look for *opportunities for the target behavior to occur*. When they see a safe behavior opportunity (SBO), they take out their checklist and complete it. If the target behavior is "safe lifting," for example, observers keep on the lookout for an SBO for lifting. They might observe such an SBO from their work station or while walking through the plant. Of course, if they see an at-risk lifting behavior and are close enough to reduce the risk, they should put their CBC aside and intervene. Intervening to reduce risk must take precedence over recording an observation of at-risk behavior.

Observing multiple behaviors

As the list of targets on a CBC increases, it becomes more and more difficult to complete a checklist from a remote location. Auditing several critical behaviors usually puts observers in close contact with another person (the performer), resulting in a one-on-one coaching situation. The observer should seek permission from the performer before recording any observations, even though a work group might have agreed on the observation process in earlier education and training meetings. If the performer wishes not to be observed, the observer should leave with no argument and a friendly smile. This helps to build the trust needed to eventually reach 100 percent participation in the DO IT process.

Multiple-behavior CBCs might be specific to a particular job or be generic in nature. The driving CBC I used with Krista was a job-specific checklist, only relevant for operating a motor vehicle. In contrast, a generic checklist is used to observe behaviors that may occur at various job sites. The CBC depicted in Figure 8.7 is generic because it is applicable to any job that requires the use of personal protective equipment (PPE). Because different PPE might be required on different jobs, certain PPE categories on the CBC may be irrelevant for some observations. For jobs requiring extra PPE, additional behaviors will be targeted on the CBC. Obviously, the observer needs to know the PPE requirements before attempting to use a CBC like the one shown in Figure 8.7.

Critical Behavior Checklist for Personal Protective Equipment

Observation period (dates): _____

Observer: _____

	TOTAL NUMBER OF EMPLOYEES OBSERVED	NUMBER OF EMPLOYEES OBSERVED USING ALL REQUIRED PPE

PPE (For Observed Area)	SAFE OBSERVATION (Proper Use of PPE)	AT-RISK OBSERVATION (Improper or No Use of PPE)
Gloves		
Safety Glasses/Shield		
Hearing Protection		
Safety Shoes		
Hard Hat		
Lifting Belt		
TOTAL		

Figure 8.7 A CBC can be used to increase the use of PPE.

The CBC in Figure 8.7 includes a place for the observer's name, but the performer's name is not recorded. Also, this CBC was designed to conduct several one-on-one behavior audits over a period of time. Each time the observer performs an observation, he or she places a checkmark in the left box (for total number of employees observed). If the performer was using all PPE required in the work area, a check would be placed in the right-hand box. From these entries, the overall percentage of safe employees can be monitored.

The checkmarks in the individual behavior categories of the CBC in Figure 8.7 are totaled and, by dividing the total number of safe checks by the total safe and at-risk checks, the percentage of safe behaviors for each PPE category can be assessed. This enables valuable feedback regarding the relative use of various devices to protect employees. Such information might suggest a need to make certain PPE more comfortable or convenient to use. It might also suggest the need for special intervention as discussed in the next three chapters.

The formula at the bottom of the CBC in Figures 8.5 and 8.6 can be used to calculate an overall percent safe score. We have found it useful to post this global score weekly for different work teams. Such social comparison information can motivate performance improvement through friendly intergroup competition. Chapter 12 also includes additional information on the design of CBCs for one-on-one behavior observation.

In conclusion

In this chapter we have gotten into the "nuts and bolts" of implementing a behavior-based safety process to develop a Total Safety Culture. The overall process is referred to as DO IT, each letter representing one of the four stages of behavior-based safety. This chapter focused on the first two stages — define and observe.

Defining critical behaviors to target for observation and intervention is not easy. A work team needs to consult a variety of sources, including the workers themselves, near-hit reports, injury records, job hazard analyses, and the plant safety director. After selecting a list of behaviors critical to preventing injuries in their work area, the team needs to struggle through defining these behaviors so precisely that all observers agree on a particular property of each behavior at least 80 percent of the time. The behavioral property most often observed for industrial safety is frequency of occurrence per individual worker or per group of employees.

A critical behavior checklist (CBC) is used to observe and record the [relative frequency of (or percentage of opportunities for) critical behaviors] throughout a work setting. If the CBC contains only a few behaviors or behavioral outcomes (conditions caused by behavior), it is possible to conduct observations without engaging in a one-on-one coaching session. This is often the best approach to use when first introducing behavior-based safety to a work culture. It is not as overwhelming or time-consuming as one-on-one coaching with a comprehensive CBC.

Over time and through building trust, a short CBC can be readily expanded and lead to one-on-one safety coaching. Safety coaching is one very effective way to implement each stage of the DO IT process and is detailed in Chapter 12. First, it is important to understand how the first two stages of DO IT can facilitate a proper behavioral analysis of the situation. This is the topic of the next chapter.

chapter nine

Behavioral safety analysis

The defining and observing processes of DO IT provide opportunities to evaluate the situational factors contributing to at-risk behavior and a possible injury. This chapter details the procedures of a behavioral safety analysis, including a step-by-step examination of the situational, social, and personal factors influencing at-risk behavior in order to determine the most cost-effective corrective action. Critical distinctions are made among four types of intervention — instruction, motivation, support, and self-management — between training and education, and between accountability and responsibility.

"A prescription without diagnosis is malpractice." — Socrates

Chapter 8 introduced the DO IT process and provided some detail about the first two steps — *define* target behavior to improve and *observe* the target behavior occurring naturally in the work environment. The CBC (critical behavior checklist) was introduced as a way to look for the occurrence of critical behaviors during a work routine and then offer workers one-on-one feedback about what was safe and what was at risk. This is behavioral coaching and is explained in more detail in Chapter 12.

While an observer is checking for safe or at-risk occurrences of critical behaviors, he or she is watching for contributing factors to at-risk behavior, as well as for the occurrence of behaviors that ought to be included on a revised CBC. The information in the "comment" section of a CBC is invaluable in determining what factors contribute to at-risk behavior and should be changed to reduce such behavior. Before intervening to correct a problem, we need to conduct a proper behavior analysis. This is the theme of this chapter. Without a careful behavioral analysis of the situation requiring intervention or corrective action, we are indeed vulnerable to accusations of malpractice.

Reducing behavioral discrepancy

It's important to consider human performance problems as a discrepancy rather than a deficiency. This places the focus on the behavior, not the individual. In other words, a difference exists between the behavior demonstrated and the behavior desired. When evaluating safety problems, this discrepancy is between behavior considered to be at-risk vs. safe.

The behavioral discrepancy could be a "sin of omission" or a "sin of substitution." The worker might have failed to perform a particular safe behavior because he or she took a short cut, or the individual could have performed a certain behavior that puts someone at risk for injury. After deciding what is safe and what is at risk for a particular individual and work situation, an action plan can be designed to reduce the discrepancy between what is and what should be. Let's consider the variety of situations or work contexts that can influence a behavioral discrepancy.

Can the task be simplified?

Before designing an intervention to reduce a behavioral discrepancy, make sure all possible engineering "fixes" have been implemented. For example, consider the many ways the environment could be changed to reduce physical effort, reach, and repetition. In other words, entertain ways to make the job more user friendly before deciding what behaviors are needed to prevent injury. This is, of course, the rationale behind ergonomics and the search for engineering solutions to occupational safety and health.

As discussed in Chapter 6, when people experience failure, as reflected by noncompliance, property damage, or personal injury, they are more likely to place blame on external than personal factors. In other words, as illustrated in Figure 9.1, people involved in an injury feel more comfortable discussing environment-related causes than individual factors. Given this self-serving bias it makes sense to begin a behavior analysis with a discussion of environmental or engineering factors. Afterward, the possibility of a constructive discussion of person factors potentially contributing to the incident increases markedly.

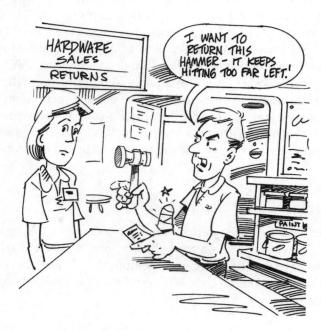

Figure 9.1 We are reluctant to accept personal responsibility for our injuries.

Sometimes behavior facilitators can be added, such as:

1. Control designs with different shapes so they can be discriminated by touch as well as sight.
2. Clear instructions placed at the point of application.
3. Color codes to aid memory and task differentiation.
4. Convenient machine lifts or conveyor rollers to help with physical jobs.

Plus, it's possible complex assignments can be redesigned to involve fewer steps or more people. To reduce boredom or repetition, simple tasks might allow for job swapping.

Ask these questions at the start of a behavior analysis:

- Can an engineering intervention make the job more user friendly?
- Can the task be redesigned to reduce physical demands?
- Can a behavior facilitator be added to improve response differentiation, reduce memory load, or increase reliability?
- Can the challenges of a complex task be shared?
- Can boring, repetitive jobs be swapped?

Is a quick fix available?

Behavior might be more at-risk than desired because expectations are unclear, resources are inadequate, or feedback is unavailable. In these cases, solutions to reducing a behavioral discrepancy are obvious and relatively inexpensive. Behavior-based instruction or demonstration can overcome invisible expectations, and behavior-based feedback can enable continuous improvement. Furthermore, a work team could decide what resources are needed to make a safe behavior more convenient, comfortable, or efficient.

When conducting this aspect of a behavioral analysis, ask these questions:

- Does the individual know what safety precautions are expected?
- Are there obvious barriers to safe work practices?
- Is the equipment as safe as possible under the circumstances?
- Is protective equipment readily available and as comfortable as possible?
- Do employees receive behavior-based feedback related to their safety?

Is safe behavior punished?

As I explained in Chapter 7, a key principle of behavior-based psychology is that behavior is motivated by its consequences. In other words, our behavior results in favorable or unfavorable consequences, and these consequences determine our future behavior. Sometimes naturally occurring consequences work against us. This is especially true in safety because safe behavior is usually less comfortable, convenient, or efficient than the at-risk alternative.

Those analyzing an incident need to try to see the situation through the eyes of the performer. This is called empathy and is illustrated in Figure 9.2. Some consequences might actually seem positive to an observer but be viewed as negative by

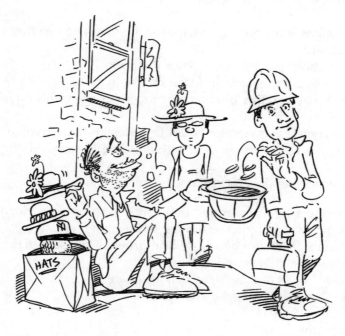

Figure 9.2 It is useful to see a situation through the eyes of the other person.

the performer. For example, a safety manager might consider an individual's public safety award a positive consequence, but for the individual it could be a negative consequence because of expected harassment from coworkers. Praise from supervisors and teachers is often overshadowed by punishing consequences from coworkers and classmates. The result is often a reduction in individual output.

In some work cultures, the interpersonal consequences for reporting an environmental hazard or near hit are more negative than positive. After all, these situations imply that someone was irresponsible or careless. It is not unusual for people to be ridiculed for wearing protective gear or using an equipment guard. It might even be considered "cool" or "macho" to work unprotected and take risky short cuts. The hidden agenda might be that "only a 'chicken' would wear that fall protection."

Mager and Pipe (1997) refer to these situations as "upside-down consequences" and suggest that whenever a behavioral discrepancy exists, part of the problem is because the desired behavior is punished. Are people put down when they should be lifted up? Are the consequences of performing well negative rather than positive, as illustrated in Figure 9.3? It's really not rare for the best performers to be "rewarded" with extra work.

Ask these questions during your behavior analysis:

- What are the consequences of desired behavior?
- Are there more negative than positive consequences of safe behavior?
- What negative consequences for safe behavior can be reduced or removed?

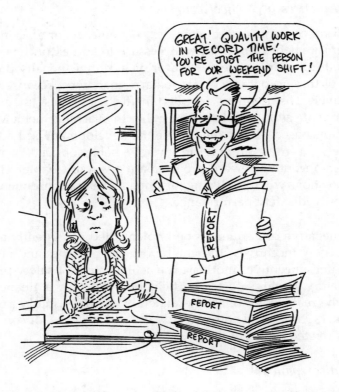

Figure 9.3 Sometimes exemplary performance is punished.

Is at-risk behavior rewarded?

As indicated previously, at-risk behavior is often followed by natural positive consequences. Short cuts are usually taken to save time and can lead to a faster rate of output. So taking an at-risk short cut can be labeled "efficient" behavior. I have analyzed several work environments, for example, where bypassing or overriding the power lockout switches was acceptable because it benefited production — the bottom line. In these cultures, the worker who could fix or adjust equipment without locking out the power was a hero. He could handle equipment problems without slowing down production.

Behavior does not occur in a vacuum. Most people perform the way they do because they expect to achieve soon, certain, and positive consequences or they expect to avoid soon, certain, and negative consequences. People take calculated risks because they expect to gain something positive or avoid something negative.

Ask these questions:

- What are the soon, certain, and positive consequences of at-risk behavior?
- Does a worker receive more attention, prestige, or status from coworkers for at-risk than safe behavior?
- What rewarding consequences of at-risk behavior can be reduced or removed?

Are extra consequences used effectively?

Because the natural consequences of comfort, convenience, or efficiency usually support at-risk over safe behavior, it's often necessary to add extra consequences. These usually take the form of incentive–reward or disincentive–penalty programs. Unfortunately, many of these programs do more harm than good because they are implemented ineffectively. Disincentives are often ineffective because they are used inconsistently and motivate avoidance behavior rather than achievement. Moreover, safety incentive programs based on outcomes stifle the development and administration of an effective safety incentive program to improve behavior. Details about designing an effective safety incentive–reward program are given in Chapter 11.

Ask these questions when analyzing the impact of extra consequences put in place to motivate improved safety performance:

- Can the negative consequences be implemented consistently and fairly?
- Can the safety incentives stifle the reporting of injuries and near misses?
- Do the safety incentives motivate the achievement of safety-process goals?
- Do monetary rewards foster participation only for a financial payoff and conceal the real benefit of safety-related behavior — injury prevention?
- Are workers recognized both individually and as teams for completing process activities related to safety improvement?

Is there a skill discrepancy?

But what about those times when the individual really does not know how to do the prescribed safe behavior? The person is "unconsciously incompetent." This situation might call for training which is a relatively expensive approach to corrective action. Most of the time a behavioral discrepancy is not caused by a genuine lack of skill. Usually people can perform the safe behavior if the conditions and the consequences are right. So training should really be the least used approach for corrective action.

Ask these questions to determine whether the behavioral discrepancy is caused by a lack of skill:

- Could the person perform the task safely if his or her life depended on it?
- Are the person's current skills adequate for the task?
- Did the person ever know how to perform the job safely?
- Has the person forgotten the safest way to perform the task?

What kind of training is needed?

Answers to the last two questions can help pinpoint the kind of intervention needed to reduce a skill discrepancy. More specifically, a "yes" answer to these questions implies the need for a skill maintenance program. Skill maintenance might be needed to help a person stay skilled — as police officers practice regularly on a pistol range to stay ready to use their guns effectively in the rare situation when they need them. This is, of course, the rationale behind periodic emergency training. People need to practice the behaviors that could prevent injury or save a life during an emergency. Fortunately, emergencies do not happen very often; but since they do not, people need to go through the motions just to "stay in practice." Then, if the infrequent event does occur, they will be ready to do the right thing.

A very different kind of situation also calls for skill maintenance training. This is when certain behaviors occur regularly, but discrepancies still exist. Contrary to circumstances requiring emergency training, this problem is not lack of practice. Rather, the person gets plenty of practice doing the behavior ineffectively or unsafely. In this case, practice does not make perfect but rather serves to entrench a bad (or at-risk) habit.

Vehicle driving behavior is perhaps the most common and relevant example of this second kind of situation in need of skill maintenance training. Most drivers know how to drive a vehicle safely, and at one time they performed very at-risk driving behaviors. However, for many drivers, safe driving has deteriorated, with some safe driving practices dropping out of some people's driving repertoire completely.

Practice with appropriate behavior-based feedback is critical for solving both types of skill discrepancies. However, if the skill is already used frequently but has deteriorated (as in the driving example), it is often necessary to add an extra feedback intervention to overpower the natural consequences that have caused the behavior to drift from the ideal.

Ask these questions to determine whether the cause of the apparent skill discrepancy is due to lack of practice or lack of feedback:

- How often is the desired skill performed?
- Does the performer receive regular feedback relevant to skill maintenance?
- How does the performer find out how well he or she is doing?

Is the person right for the job?

From this discussion it is clear a skill discrepancy can be handled in one of two ways. Change the job or change the behavior. The first approach is exemplified by simplifying the task, while the latter approach is reflected in practice and behavior-based feedback or behavioral coaching. But what if a person's interests, skills, or prior experiences are incompatible with the job?

Ask these questions to determine whether the individual has the potential to handle the job safely and effectively:

- Does the person have the physical capability to perform as desired?
- Does the person have the mental capability to handle the complexities of the task?
- Is the person overqualified for the job and, thus, prone to boredom or dissatisfaction?
- Can the person learn how to do the job as desired?

In summary

Figure 9.4 summarizes the main steps of a behavior-based incident analysis with a flow chart of ten basic questions to ask. Before an individual worker is targeted with a training intervention, engineering strategies are considered for task simplification, and a number of other issues should be addressed.

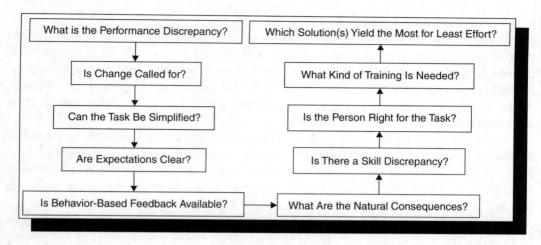

Figure 9.4 Ask ten basic questions to conduct a behavior-based incident analysis.

The bottom line: Before deciding on an intervention approach, conduct a careful analysis of the situation, the behavior, and the individual(s) involved in an observed discrepancy between desired and actual behavior. Do not impulsively assume corrective action to improve behavior requires training or "discipline." A behavioral incident analysis will likely give priority to a number of alternative intervention approaches. I discuss critical disadvantages of using "discipline" or a punishment approach to corrective action in Chapter 11.

Behavior-based safety training

The principles and procedures of behavior-based safety, including behavioral observation and interpersonal coaching, are new to most people. Therefore, to achieve a Total Safety Culture, behavior-based safety training is needed throughout a work culture. Everyone in a work force needs to understand the basic rationale or theory behind the behavior-based approach. Then work teams need to participate in exercises to customize observation, analysis, and feedback procedures for their work areas. Finally, practice sessions are needed in which individuals and teams receive supportive and corrective feedback regarding their implementation of behavior-based safety — from designing a CBC and analyzing CBC results to using a CBC for constructive intervention.

Why should employees want such training? First, as I've indicated in earlier chapters, behavior-based safety works to reduce injuries. The principles and methods of behavior-based safety are applicable in many situations — whenever and wherever human performance is a factor and can be improved. Thus, training in behavior-based safety provides skills useful in numerous domains at work, at home, during recreational and sport activities, and traveling in between.

While people need sufficient training to feel confident they can complete a certain task, they also need to believe the job is worthwhile. This requires education, not training. There's a difference. Actually, you already know the distinction. Do you want your teenager to receive sex education or sex training? In contrast, are you satisfied if your teenager receives only "driver education," or do you prefer some "training" with that education?

Because people know intuitively the difference between education and training, misusing these terms can lead to problems. We might perceive safety training as a step-by-step procedure or program with no room for individual creativity, ownership, or empowerment. This is how safety can come to be viewed as a top-down "flavor of the month." If we do not educate people about the principles or rationale behind a particular safety policy, program, or process, they might participate only minimally. They will perceive the program as a requirement rather than an opportunity to make a difference.

By the same token, safety education without follow-up training will not reap optimal benefits. Learning the theory or principles behind an intervention approach is crucial for customizing intervention procedures for a particular work situation, but after the procedures are developed — with input from an educated work team — training is necessary. People need to know precisely what to do. With proper education, these participants can refine or upgrade procedures when appropriate; with a change in procedures, additional training is obviously needed.

Bottom line: People need both education and training to improve. As Deming is known for reiterating at his quality and productivity workshops, "There's no substitute for knowledge" (Deming, 1991, 1992). Indeed, without gaining profound knowledge through education and training, we are like the clown in Figure 9.5. We do our best with what we now know. We use our biased and ineffective common sense.

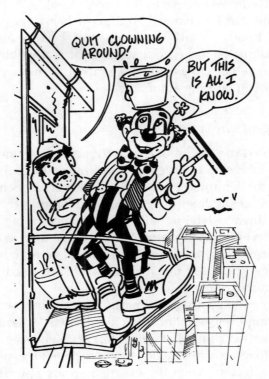

Figure 9.5 Without education and training, we clown around
with our biased common sense.

Intervention and the flow of behavior change

Taken together, education and training are instruction, and instruction represents a type of intervention. Under certain circumstances, instruction is sufficient to change behavior. Sometimes instruction does not work, and another type of intervention is needed. Perhaps a motivational intervention is called for, or maybe only supportive intervention is needed. A complete behavioral safety analysis should often include a recommendation for a certain type of behavior-change intervention. This section provides information critical for making such a recommendation. Then subsequent chapters provide guidance for designing a certain type of behavior-change intervention.

Three types of behavior

On-the-job behavior starts out as other-directed behavior, in the sense that we follow someone else's instructions. Such direction can come from a training program, an operation manual, or policy statement. After learning what to do, essentially by memorizing or internalizing the appropriate instructions, our behavior can become self-directed. We can talk to ourselves or formulate an image before performing a behavior in order to activate the right response.

Performed frequently and consistently over a period of time, some behaviors become automatic. A habit is formed. Some habits are good and some are not good, depending on their short- and long-term consequences. If implemented correctly, rewards, recognition, and other positive consequences can facilitate the transfer of behavior from the self-directed phase to the habit phase.

Before a bad habit can be changed to a good habit, the target behavior must become self-directed. In other words, people need to become aware of their undesirable habit (as in at-risk behavior) before adjustment is possible. Then, if people are motivated to improve (perhaps as a result of an incentive–reward program), their new self-directed behavior can become automatic.

Three kinds of intervention strategies

In Chapter 8, I explained the ABC model as a framework to understand and analyze behavior as well as to develop interventions for improving behavior. Recall that the "A" stands for activators or antecedent events that precede behavior ("B"), and "C" refers to the consequences following behavior and produced by it. Of course, you remember activators direct behavior, while consequences motivate behavior.

Instructional intervention. An instructional intervention is typically an activator or antecedent event used to get new behavior started or to move behavior from the automatic (habit) stage to the self-directed stage. Or it is used to improve behavior already in the self-directed stage.

This type of intervention consists primarily of activators, as exemplified by education sessions, training exercises, and directive feedback. Because your purpose is to instruct, the intervention comes before the target behavior and focuses on helping the performer internalize your instructions. As we have all experienced, this type of intervention is more effective when the instructions are specific and given one-on-one. Role playing exercises provide instructors opportunities to customize directions specific to individual attempts to improve. They also allow participants the chance to receive rewarding feedback for their improvement.

Supportive intervention. Once a person learns the right way to do something, practice is important so the behavior becomes part of a natural routine. Continued practice leads to fluency and, in many cases, to automatic or habitual behavior. This is an especially desirable state for safety-related behavior, but practice does not come easily and benefits greatly from supportive intervention. We need support to reassure us we are doing the right thing and to encourage us to keep going.

While instructional intervention consists primarily of activators, supportive intervention focuses on the application of positive consequences. Thus, when we give people rewarding feedback or recognition for particular safe behavior, we are showing our appreciation for their efforts and increasing the likelihood they will perform the behavior again. Each occurrence of the desired behavior facilitates fluency and helps build a good habit.

Motivational intervention. When people know what to do but do not do it, a motivational intervention is needed. In other words, they require some external encouragement or pressure to change. Instruction alone is obviously insufficient because they are knowingly doing the wrong thing. As I discussed in Chapter 4, we refer to this as taking a calculated risk.

We usually perform calculated risks because we perceive the positive consequences of the at-risk behavior to be more powerful than the negative consequences. This is because the positive consequences of comfort, convenience, and efficiency are immediate and certain, while the negative consequence of at-risk behavior (such as an injury) is improbable and seems remote. Furthermore, the safe alternative is relatively inconvenient, uncomfortable, or inefficient, and these negative consequences are immediate and certain.

This is when an incentive–reward program is useful. Such a program attempts to motivate a certain target behavior by promising people a positive consequence if they perform it. The promise is the incentive and the consequence is the reward. In safety, this kind of motivational intervention is much less common than a disincentive–penalty program. This is when a rule, policy, or law threatens to give people a negative consequence (a penalty) if they fail to comply or take a calculated risk.

The flow of behavior change

Figure 9.6 reviews this intervention information by depicting relationships among four competency states (unconscious incompetence, conscious incompetence, conscious competence, and unconscious competence) and four intervention approaches (instructional intervention, motivational intervention, supportive intervention, and self-management). When people are unaware of the safe work practice (i.e., they are unconsciously incompetent), they need repeated instructional intervention until they understand what to do. Then, as depicted on the left-hand side of Figure 9.6, the critical question is whether they perform the desired behavior. If they do, the question of behavioral fluency is relevant. A fluent response becomes a habit or part of a regular routine, and thus the individual is unconsciously competent.

When workers know how to perform a task safely but do not, they are considered consciously incompetent or irresponsible. This is when an external motivational

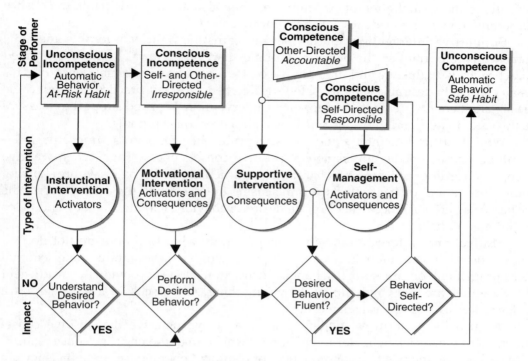

Figure 9.6 Awareness (conscious vs. unconscious) and safety-related behavior (competence vs. incompetence) determine which of four types of interventions is relevant.

intervention can be useful, as discussed previously. Then when the desired behavior occurs at least once, supportive intervention is needed to get the behavior to a fluent state. Techniques for giving supportive recognition are described in Chapter 12.

Most people need supportive intervention for their safe behavior. In other words, most experienced workers know what to do in order to prevent injury on their jobs and have performed their jobs safely one or more times, but the safe way might not be habitual. The individual is consciously competent but needs supportive recognition or feedback for response maintenance and increased fluency.

Figure 9.6 illustrates a distinction between conscious competence/other-directed and conscious competence/self-directed. If a safe work practice is self-directed, the employee is considered responsible and a self-management intervention is relevant. As detailed elsewhere (Geller, 1998a; Watson and Tharp, 1997), the methods and tools of effective self-management are derived from behavioral science research and are perfectly consistent with the principles of behavior-based safety.

In essence, self-management involves the application of the DO IT process introduced in Chapter 8 to one's own behavior. This means:

1. Defining one or more target behavior(s) to improve
2. Monitoring these behaviors
3. Manipulating relevant activators and consequences to increase desired behavior and decrease undesired behavior
4. Tracking continual change in the target behavior(s) in order to determine the impact of the self-management process

Accountability vs. responsibility

From the perspective of large-scale safety and health promotion, the distinction in Figure 9.6 between accountable and responsible is critical. People often use the words accountability and responsibility interchangeably. Whether you hold someone accountable or responsible for getting something done, you mean the same thing. You want that person to accomplish a certain task and you intend on making sure it happens. However, let us consider the receiving end of this situation. How does a person feel about an assignment — does he or she feel accountable or responsible? Here is where a difference is evident.

When you are held accountable, you are asked to reach a certain objective or goal, often within a designated time period. However, you might not feel responsible to meet the deadline, or you might feel responsible enough to complete the assignment, but that's all. You do only what is required and no more. In this case, accountability is the same as responsibility.

There are times, however, when you extend your responsibility beyond accountability. You do more than what's required. You go beyond the call of duty as defined by a particular accountability system. This is often essential when it comes to industrial safety and health. To improve safety beyond the current performance plateau experienced by many companies, workers need to extend their responsibility for safety beyond that for which they are held accountable. They need to transition from an other-directed state to a self-directed state.

Many jobs are accomplished by a lone worker. There's no supervisor or coworker around to hold the employee accountable for performing the job safely. The challenge for safety professionals and corporate leaders is to build the kind of work culture that enables or facilitates responsibility or self-accountability for safety. I cover ways to make this happen in Part 5, especially Chapter 16.

In conclusion

This chapter offered some basic guidelines for diagnosing the human behavior aspects of a safety-related problem. Many situational, social, and individual factors contribute to a behavioral discrepancy — a distinction between the behavior performed and the behavior desired. In safety terms, this is the difference between at-risk and safe behavior.

Most of the factors contributing to a behavioral discrepancy are due to the context in which the task is performed or characteristics of the task itself. Common contextual variables include:

1. Unclear or misunderstood expectancies
2. Upside-down contingencies that reward at-risk behavior or punish safe behavior
3. The lack of behavior-based feedback to help people improve

Often a job can be simplified or re-engineered to reduce physical or mental effort, which decreases the probability of personal injury.

Training should be considered only after critical contextual and task variables have been analyzed and corrected. It's usually a good idea to include some education with the training, meaning relevant theory, principles, and rationale are presented to justify the step-by-step procedures taught and practiced. Adequate education also enables worker customization of procedures to fit a particular work context. This, in turn, leads to employee ownership of the process, feelings of responsibility, and increased involvement.

Education and training reflect an instructional approach to corrective action. This type of intervention is obviously most effective when the participants are willing to learn. They are unaware of the correct procedures and are "unconsciously incompetent." Instruction will not help much for people who know what to do but do not do it. These individuals are "consciously incompetent" and need a motivational intervention, as discussed in Chapter 11.

For most employees, the issue is not a matter of knowing what is safe. They periodically perform all of the safe operating procedures called for on the job. The problem is consistency or fluency. They do not follow the safe protocol every time. These people need supportive intervention to keep them safe, as discussed in Chapter 13.

When safe work practices are relatively convenient, like putting on PPE or buckling a safety belt, the behavior can become habitual. When such behavior becomes a natural part of the work routine, the participant is considered "unconsciously competent." However, some behaviors, like locking out a power source, are relatively complex and never reach the automatic stage. Regular supportive intervention is often needed to keep these inconvenient behaviors going, unless the individual is self-directed with regard to the particular behavior.

Self-directed individuals hold themselves accountable for doing the right thing, even when the behavior is relatively uncomfortable and inconvenient. These people certainly appreciate supportive intervention from managers, friends, and coworkers, but they keep performing the safe behavior when no one is around to support them. These self-directed workers hold themselves accountable. They feel responsible and go beyond the call of duty to prevent injuries to themselves and others. I call this "actively caring" — the focus throughout Part 5 of this book.

part four

Behavior-based intervention

chapter ten

Intervening with activators

Intervention techniques to increase safe behaviors or decrease at-risk behaviors are either activators or consequences. This chapter explains activators, with real-world examples showing how to develop effective strategies. This discussion is framed by six principles for maximizing the impact of activators.

"Best efforts are not enough, you have to know what to do." — W. Edwards Deming

In Chapter 9, I showed how the activator–behavior–consequence (ABC) model can be used to diagnose the contributing factors to an incident or at-risk behavior and to decide on a plan for corrective action. With this chapter, we begin our discussion of intervention design and implementation to improve safety-related behavior. As such, the ABC model is used as introduced in Chapter 8 — as a framework for designing behavior-change interventions.

First, let me reiterate the need for safety interventions. As I've said before, maintaining our own safe behavior is not easy. It's usually one long fight with human nature, because in most situations activators and consequences naturally support risky behavior in lieu of safe behavior. At-risk behavior often allows for more immediate fun, comfort, and convenience than safe behavior, prompting the need for special intervention to direct and motivate safe behavior. Activators are generally much easier and less expensive to use than consequences, so it's not surprising they are employed much more often to promote safe behavior. Posters or signs are perhaps the most popular activators for safety.

- Some bear only a general message — Safety is a Condition of Employment; others refer to a specific behavior — Hard Hat Required in This Area.
- Some signs request the occurrence of a behavior — Walk, Wear Ear Plugs in This Area; others want you to avoid a certain behavior — Don't Walk, No Smoking Area.
- Sometimes a relatively convenient response is requested — Buckle-Up, while other signs prompt relatively inconvenient behaviors — Lock Out All Energy Sources Before Repairing Equipment.
- Some signs imply consequences — Use Eye Protection: Don't Be Blinded by the Light; others do not — Wear Safety Goggles.
- We might be reminded of a general purpose — Actively Care for a Total Safety Culture, or challenged — 100 Percent Safe Behavior is Our Goal This Year.

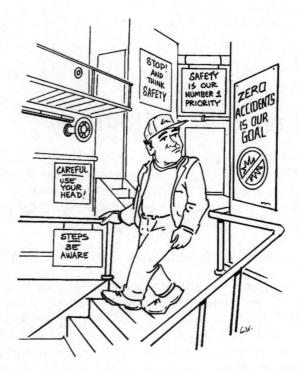

Figre 10.1 Safety activators can be overwhelming and ineffective.

I have visited a number of work environments where all of these types of safety signs were displayed. In fact, I have seen situations that make the illustration in Figure 10.1 seem not very far fetched. Does this sort of "over-kill" work to change behavior and reduce injuries? If you answered "no," then this time your common sense was correct because you have been there and experienced the ineffectiveness of many safety signs.

Which signs would you eliminate from Figure 10.1? How would you change certain signs to increase their impact? What activator strategies would you use instead of the signs? This chapter enables you to answer these questions — not on the basis of common sense but from behavioral science research.

Let's consider six key principles for increasing the impact of activators.

Principle #1: Specify behavior

Figure 10.2 illustrates "explosively" the need to include sufficient response information with a behavioral request, but too much specificity can bury a message, as illustrated in Figure 10.3. Activators ought to specify a desired response, but not overwhelm with complexity, as I have seen in a number of industrial signs. Overly complex signs are easy to overlook — with time they just blend into the wood-work. Keeping signs salient or noticeable is clearly a challenge.

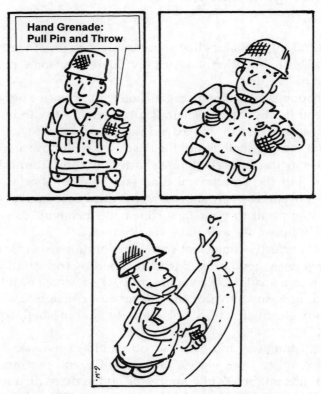

Figure 10.2 Some activators are not specific enough.

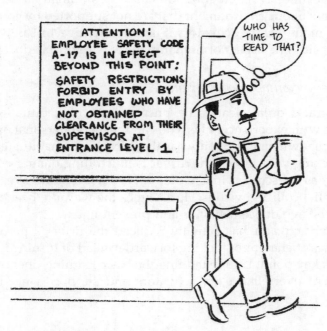

Figure 10.3 Some signs are too complex to be effective.

Principle #2: Maintain salience with novelty

Habituation

It is perfectly natural for activators like sign messages to lose their impact over time. This process is called habituation, and it's considered by some psychologists to be the simplest form of learning.

Habituation happens even among organisms with primitive nervous systems. For example, when you lightly tap the shell of a large snail it withdraws into its shell. After about 30 seconds the snail will extend its body from the shell and continue on its way. When you tap the shell again, the snail will withdraw again. However, this time the snail will stay inside its shell for a shorter duration. Your third tap will cause withdrawal again, but the withdrawal time will be even shorter. Each tap on the snail's shell results in successively shorter withdrawal time until eventually the snail will stop responding at all to your tap. The snail's behavior of withdrawal to the activator — shell tapping — will have habituated.

Habituation is perfectly consistent with an evolutionary perspective. If there is no obvious consequence (good or bad) from responding to a stimulus, the organism, be it an employee or a snail, stops reacting to it. It's a waste of time and energy to continue responding to an activator that seems to be insignificant. What would a snail do in a rain storm if it did not learn to ignore shell taps that have no consequence?

Consider the distractions and distress you would experience daily if you could not learn to ignore noises from voices, radios, traffic, and machinery. At first these environmental sounds might be quite noticeable and perhaps distracting, but through habituation they become insignificant background noise. They no longer divert attention nor interfere with ongoing performance.

What's the relevance of habituation for safety? It's human nature to habituate to everyday activators in our environment that are not supported by consequences. This is the case with many safety activators. Staying attentive to safety activators is a continuous fight with one aspect of human nature — habituation.

Warning beepers: a common work example

Figure 10.4 illustrates quite clearly the phenomenon of habituation and reduced activator salience with experience. I bet you can reflect on personal experiences quite similar to the one shown here. Not only has the brick mason habituated to the familiar "beep" of the backing vehicle, but the driver is illustrating danger compensation (or risk homeostasis) as I discussed in Chapter 6. He's not looking over his shoulder to check for a potential collision victim. He assumes the warning beeper is sufficient to activate coworkers' avoidance behavior and prevent injury.

This particular activator has actually reduced the driver's perceived risk. This influences his at-risk behavior of looking forward instead of turning his head to check his blind spots. A key point: Understanding the basic learning phenomenon of habituation can prevent overreliance on activators and support a need to work more defensively.

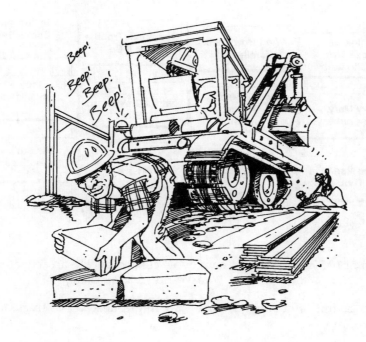

Figure 10.4 Some signals we rely on lose impact over time.

Principle #3: Vary the message

What does habituation tell us about the design of safety activators? Essentially, we need to vary the message. When an activator changes it can become more salient and noticeable. The "safety share" discussed in Chapter 7 follows this principle. When participants in a group meeting are asked to share something they have done for safety since the last meeting, the examples will vary considerably. Similarly, group discussions of near hits and potential corrective actions will also vary dramatically. The messages from safety shares and near-hit discussions are also salient because they are personal, genuine, and distinct.

Changeable signs

Over the years I've noticed a variety of techniques for changing the message on safety signs. There are removable slats to place different messages. I'm sure most of you have seen computer-generated signs with an infinite variety of safety messages. Some plants even have video screens in break rooms, lunch rooms, visitor lounges, and hallways that display many kinds of safety messages, conveniently controlled by user friendly computer software.

Who determines the content of these messages? I know who should — the target audience for these signs. The people expected to follow the specific behavioral advice should have as much input as possible in defining message content. Many organizations can get suggestions for safety messages just by asking. But if employees are not

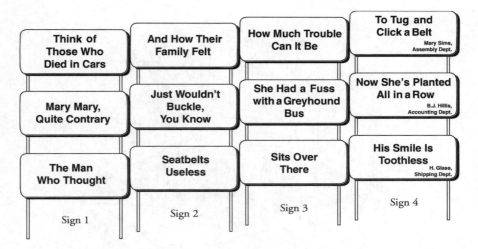

Figure 10.5 In 1986, Ford employees created buckle-up activators
for display at Ford World Headquarters.

accustomed to giving safety suggestions, they might need a positive consequence to
motivate their input.

Worker-designed safety slogans

Here's what I'm talking about. In 1985, employees and visitors driving into the main
parking lot for Ford World Headquarters in Dearborn, MI, passed a series of four
signs arranged with sequential messages, like the old Burma Shave signs. The messages were rotated periodically from a pool of 55 employee entries in a limerick contest
for safety-belt promotion. My three favorites are illustrated in Figure 10.5.

Notice that the last sign in each series of safety-belt promotion messages includes
the name and department of the author. This public recognition, with the author's
permission, of course, provides a positive consequence or reward to the participant.
It also reminds all sign viewers that many different people from various work areas
are actively involved in safety. Through positive recognition and observational learning, including vicarious reinforcement, this simple technique promotes ownership
and involvement in a safety process. This leads to the next principle.

Principle #4: Involve the target audience

Figure 10.6 depicts a sample promise card for involving people in making a commitment to perform a particular behavior. The target behavior to increase in frequency
could be selected by a safety director, group leader, or through a group consensus
discussion. This behavior is written on the promise card, perhaps by each individual
in a group. Group members decide on the duration of the promise period and write
the end date on the card. Then each group member should be encouraged, not coerced,
to sign and date a card. I have found this group application of the safe behavior
promise strengthens a sense of group cohesion or belonging. Follow these procedural
points for optimal results:

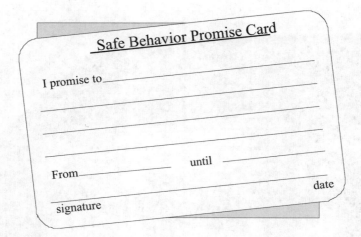

Figure 10.6 A promise card activates a behavioral commitment.

- Define the desired target behavior specifically.
- Involve the group in discussing the personal and group value of the target behavior.
- Make the commitment for a specified period of time that is challenging but not overwhelming.
- Assure everyone that signing the card is only a personal commitment, not a company contract.
- There should be no penalties (not even criticism) for breaking a promise.
- Encourage everyone to sign the card, but do not use pressure tactics.
- Signers should keep their promise cards in their possession, or post them in their work areas as reminders.

The more involvement and personal choice solicited during the completion of this activator strategy, the better each individual feels about the process. Personal commitment to perform a specific behavior is activated as a result; those involved in the process should feel obligated to fulfill the promise. Signing the card publicly in a group meeting also implicates social consequences to motivate compliance. That is, many participants will be motivated to keep their promise to avoid disapproval from a group member. When individuals keep their promise, recognition and approval from the group reinforces and supports maintenance of the targeted safe behavior.

The "Flash for Life"

The second activator intervention I want to relate dates back to 1984, when I developed the "Flash for Life." Here's how it works. A person displays to vehicle occupants the front side of an 11- by 14-inch flash card that reads, "Please Buckle Up — I Care." If someone buckles up after viewing this message, the "flasher" flips the card over to display the bold words, "Thank You For Buckling Up."

For the first evaluation of this behavior change intervention, the "flasher" was in the front seat of a stopped vehicle and the "flashee" was the driver of an adjacent,

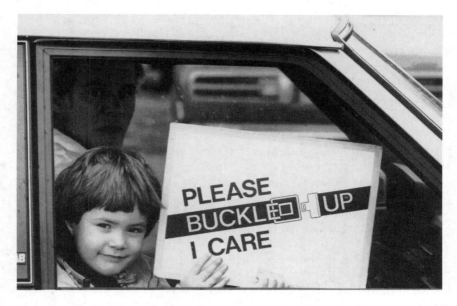

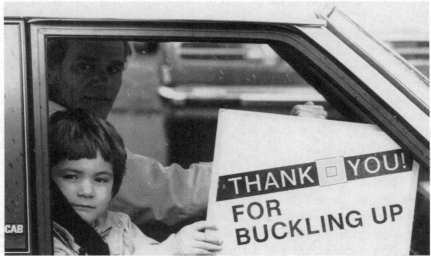

Figure 10.7 *Top:* My daughter Karly "flashes" drivers to buckle up in 1984. *Bottom:* When the driver buckles up, Karly flips over the flash card to give positive consequence.

stopped vehicle. The flash card was shown to 1087 unbuckled drivers, and of the 82 percent who looked at the card, 22 percent complied immediately with the buckle-up request.

My younger daughter, Karly, was the "flasher" for about 30 percent of the trials in this study. As shown in Figure 10.7, Karly was only three and one-half years of age at the time. On a few occasions we got a hand signal that was not used to indicate a right or left turn. Once Karly asked, "Daddy, what does that mean?" and I answered, "It means you're number one, honey; they're just using the wrong finger."

When hearing about this Flash for Life project, many of my colleagues expressed concern for my sanity. "Why do you waste your time?" some would say. "Getting 22 percent to buckle up is not a big deal, and most of those who buckled up for your daughter only did it the one time. They probably won't buckle up the next day."

I had two answers to this sort of pessimism. First, achievement is built on "small wins." People need to break up big problems or challenges into small, achievable steps, and then work on each successive step, one at a time. We cannot expect to solve a major safety problem like low use of PPE with one intervention technique, but we need to start somewhere. If everyone contributed a "small win" for safety, the cumulative effects could be tremendous.

My second reply focused on the powerful influence of involvement. This intervention procedure enabled my young daughter to get involved in a safety project, even though she did not yet understand the concept of "safety." Every time she "flashed" another person to buckle up, her own commitment to practice the target behavior increased. I never had to remind her to use her safety belt.

The "Airline Lifesaver"

My third personal experience with an activator intervention is one I have used since November 1984, whenever boarding a commercial airplane. I hand the flight attendant a 3- by 5-inch "Airline Lifesaver" card. The card indicates that airlines have been the most effective promoters of seat-belt use and requests that someone in the flight crew make the following announcement: "Now that you have worn a seat belt for the safest part of your trip, the flight crew would like to remind you to buckle up during your ground transportation."

From November 1984 to May 2001, I distributed the Airline Lifesaver on 1050 flights, and on more than 40 percent of these occasions the flight attendant gave a public buckle-up reminder.

Many friends have laughed at the Airline Lifesaver, claiming I'm wasting my time. A common comment was "No one listens to the airline announcements anyway, and besides, do you really think an airline message could be enough to motivate people to buckle up if they don't already?"

Ah, but consider this personal experience from the mid-1980s. I observed a woman approach the driver of an airport shuttle, asking her, "Please use your safety belt." The driver immediately buckled up. When I thanked the woman for making the buckle-up request, she replied that she normally would not be so assertive but she had just heard a buckle-up reminder on her flight, "and if a stewardess can request safety-belt use, so can I."

Except for a few anecdotes like this one, it's impossible to assess the direct buckle-up influence of the Airline Lifesaver. However, it's "safe" to assume that the beneficial, large-scale impact of this activator is a direct function of the number of individuals who deliver the reminder card to airline personnel. If the delivery of an Airline Lifesaver does not influence a single airline passenger to use a safety belt during ground transportation, at least the act of handing an Airline Lifesaver card to another person should increase the card deliverer's commitment to personal safety-belt use.

Of course, the primary purpose of getting involved in a safety intervention is to prevent injury or improve a person's quality of life. Unfortunately, we rarely see these most important consequences. Thus, we need motivation, feedback, interpersonal approval, and self-talk. We tell ourselves the safe behavior is "the right thing to do,"

THANKS!!!   On December 11, 1994 I was a passenger on Flt. 499 from Houston to San Francisco. At the end of the flight the pilot came on the speaker and said: "Now that the safest part of your journey is over and you are about to make the most dangerous part of your journey, please remember to use your seat belt...." I may have the words a little off, but I think you know the message. This was the second time I heard the message. The first was at the ASSE PDC in Dallas.

I am an obsessive seat belt user but when I got into the taxi, the seat belt was, as usual, buried in the seat. Usually when I find this in a cab I say, "the heck with it," but I can honestly say the pilot's message motivated me and I "dug out" the seat belt.

At over 70 mph the taxi hydroplaned and struck the guardrail. Thank God for the new barriers that prevent cars from being thrown back onto traffic. Thank you and the pilot for the reminder. My wife and children are also grateful. I suffered a neck and shoulder injury – I think it is relatively minor. It could have been much worse. I should mention the driver was O.K. He was wearing his seat belt.

In safety it is seldom we can point to a particular event we can take credit for. This is one for you. Thanks again.

Figure 10.8 I received these words of encouragement from Steven Boydston on December 28, 1994.

and that someday an injury will be prevented. We cannot count the number of injuries we prevent; we just need to "keep the faith."

On December 28, 1994, I received a special letter from Steven Boydston, then assistant vice president of Alexander & Alexander of Texas, Inc., which helps me "keep the faith" that the Airline Lifesaver makes a difference. The encouraging words in this letter are repeated in Figure 10.8. This success story is itself an activator for such proactive interventions as the Airline Lifesaver. It sure worked for me.

Principle #5: Activate close to response opportunity

Most of the effective activators discussed so far occurred at the time and place the target behavior should happen. The Flash-for-Life card was presented when people were in their vehicles and could readily buckle up, and I give airline attendants the Airline Lifesaver card when boarding the plane. Actually, I believe I would get more compliance with the request for a buckle-up announcement if I handed an attendant the announcement card at the end of the flight — closer to the opportunity to make the requested response. In fact, when I inquire about the lack of a buckle-up announcement while deplaning, the most common excuse is "I forgot."

Buckle-up road signs

Over a two-year period my students evaluated the behavioral impact of buckle-up activators located along the road in my hometown of Newport — a small rural

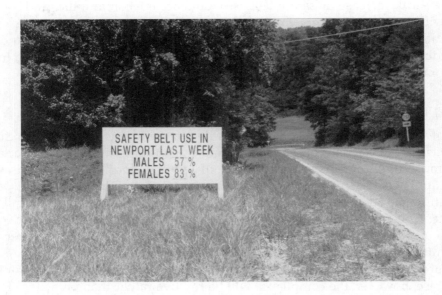

Figure 10.9 The feedback sign in Newport, VA, compared the safety-belt use
of males and females.

community in southwest Virginia. They started collecting baseline data in March
1993, by unobtrusively observing and recording the safety-belt use of vehicle drivers
and passengers from a parked vehicle near the intersection of a four-lane highway
(Highway 460) and the two-lane road (Route 42) leading into Newport. Observations
were taken of vehicles entering or leaving Route 42 to Newport, as well as vehicles
continuing on Highway 460, during most weekdays from approximately 4:00 to 6:30
p.m., when the Newport traffic was heaviest.

After 13 weeks of baseline observation, the sign shown in Figure 10.9 was positioned approximately 7 feet from Route 42 and 300 feet from the intersection of Route
42 and Highway 460. The sign was eight feet long by four feet high, and the buckle-
up message shown in Figure 10.9 was painted on both sides in black eight-inch-high
letters against a white background. The sign could not be seen by occupants of vehicles
continuing along Highway 460.

Vehicle observations continued for 24 weeks, then the feedback sign was removed.
After 21 weeks of observation during this withdrawal condition, the signs were
reinstated, but with a different message. We wanted to see if safety-belt use could be
activated with a sign that did not need to be changed weekly to reflect belt-use
feedback. The new message was "We buckle up in Newport to set an example for our
children." Note that this message specifies an actively caring consequence for the
requested behavior. We continued to record safety belt use for 19 more weeks while
this new buckle-up activator was in place.

The results of our long-term field observations showed quite clearly that both
signs increased safety-belt use substantially. While mean safety-belt use in vehicles
traveling on Highway 460 remained relatively stable, the mean safety-belt use in
vehicles entering or exiting the road on which the signs were placed increased almost
30 percent with placement and removal of the buckle-up activators. This suggests

that large-scale increases in safety-belt use would occur if communities and companies nationwide implemented this simple activator intervention. Our findings also suggest that an activator message referring to actively caring consequences can be as effective as a feedback sign that requires more effort to implement because of the need to collect behavioral data and post weekly feedback.

Principle #6: Implicate consequences

Many of the successful activator strategies illustrated in this chapter were explicitly or implicitly connected to consequences. Signing a promise card or public declaration, for example, implicates social approval vs. disapproval for honoring vs. disavowing a commitment. Consequences motivated employees to create safety slogans, and the most influential activators usually made reference to consequences. In a similar vein, the salient beep of a radar detector effectively motivates reduced vehicle speeds because it enables drivers to avoid a negative consequence — an encounter with a police officer.

Figure 10.10 illustrates the influence of negative consequences on activator impact. In this case, however, the compliance will be reactive rather than proactive. That is, a negative incident occurred because the specific behavior-focused instructions were not followed. From now on, however, it's likely this activator will be effective for this person. And if he shares the negative incident and its messy consequences with other store personnel, this activator will take on increased significance and behavioral impact.

Incentives vs. disincentives

Activators that signal the availability of a consequence are either incentives or disincentives. An *incentive* announces to an individual or group, in written or oral form, the availability of a reward. This pleasant consequence follows the occurrence of a certain behavior or an outcome of one or more behaviors. In contrast, a *disincentive* is an activator announcing or signaling the possibility of receiving a penalty. This unpleasant consequence is contingent on the occurrence of a particular undesirable behavior.

The next chapter discusses how to design and apply consequences to motivate behavior. At this point, it's important to understand that the *power of an activator to motivate behavior depends on the consequence it signals.* Figure 10.11 illustrates this connection between activator and consequence. If a sign like the one shown in Figure 10.11 motivated a driver to attempt safer driving practices, it would work because of the potential consequences implied by the activator. Every time the driver got into the vehicle, she would be reminded of potential consequences for certain driving practices. Incidentally, do you perceive the sign on the vehicle in Figure 10.11 as an incentive or disincentive?

My guess is you perceived it as a disincentive rather than an incentive. I bet you saw the sign as a threat to reduce at-risk driving, rather than an incentive to encourage safe driving. You would not expect dad to get a phone call commending his daughter's driving. If any phone calls were made, they would be to criticize at-risk or discourteous driving. This is exactly how my daughter, Krista, perceived the activator in Figure 10.11. As the illustration suggests, she flatly refused to drive with such a sign on our car.

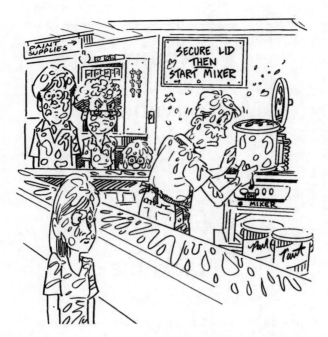

Figure 10.10 Negative consequences can increase the subsequent impact of an activator.

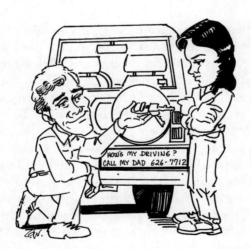

Figure 10.11 The most powerful activators imply immediate consequences.

Setting goals for consequences

Let's talk about safety goals in the context of activators that imply consequences. Dr. Deming told us to "eliminate slogans, exhortations, and targets for the work force . . . eliminate work standards . . . management by objectives, and management by the numbers" (Deming, 1985). Does this mean we should stop setting safety objectives and goals? Should we stop trying to activate safe behaviors with

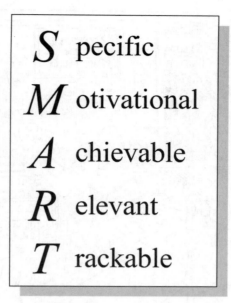

Figure 10.12   SMART goals are effective activators.

signs, slogans, and goal statements? Does this mean we should stop counting OSHA recordables and lost-time cases, and stop holding people accountable for their work injuries?

Answers to all of these questions are "yes," if you take Deming's points literally. However, my evaluation of Deming's scholarship and workshop presentations, and my personal communications with him in 1990 and 1991, have led me to believe that Deming meant we should eliminate goal setting, slogans, and work targets as they are currently implemented. Deming was not criticizing *appropriate* use of goal setting, management by objectives, and activators; rather he was lamenting the frequent incorrect use of these activator interventions.

Set SMART goals. I remember the techniques for setting effective goals with the acronym SMART, as illustrated in Figure 10.12. SMART goal setting defines what will happen when the goal is reached (the consequences), and tracks progress toward achieving the goal. Rewarding feedback for completing intermediate steps toward the ultimate goal is a consequence that motivates continued progress. Of course, it's critical that the people asked to work toward the goal "buy in" or believe in the goal. They must believe the goal is relevant to achieving a worthwhile consequence and that they have the skills and resources to achieve it.

Focus on the process. Safety goals should focus on process activities that can contribute to injury prevention. Workers need to discuss what they can do to reduce injuries, from reporting and analyzing near hits to conducting safety audits of environmental conditions and work practices. One safety steering committee I worked with wanted to increase daily interpersonal communications regarding safety. They set a goal for their group to achieve 500 safety communications within the following month. To do this, they had to develop a system for tracking and recording "safety talk." They designed a wallet-sized "SMART Card" for recording their interactions with others about safety. One member of the group volunteered to tally and graph the daily card totals.

Another work group I consulted with set a goal of 300 behavioral observations of lifting. Employees had agreed to observe each other's lifting behaviors according to a critical behavior checklist they had developed. If each worker completed an average of one lifting observation per day, the group would reach their goal within the month. Each of these work groups reached their safety goals within the expected time period, and as a result they celebrated their "small win" at a group luncheon.

These two examples illustrate the use of SMART goals and depict safety as process-focused and achievement-oriented, rather than the standard and less effective outcome-focused and failure-oriented approach promoted by injury-based goals. More important, these goals were employee driven. Workers were motivated to initiate the safety process because it was their idea. They got involved in the process and owned it. And they stayed motivated because the SMART goals were like a roadmap telling them where they were going, when they would get there, and how to follow their progress along the way.

In conclusion

In this chapter, I have presented examples of intervention techniques called activators. They occur before desired or undesired behavior to direct potential performers. Based on rigorous behavioral science research and backed by real-world examples, six principles for maximizing effective activators were given:

- Specify behavior.
- Maintain salience with novelty.
- Vary the message.
- Involve the target audience.
- Activate close to response opportunity.
- Implicate consequences.

We are constantly bombarded with activators. At home we get telephone solicitations, junk mail, television commercials, and verbal requests from family members. At work, it's phone mail, e-mail, memos, policy pronouncements, and verbal directions from supervisors and coworkers. On the road, there's no escape from billboards, traffic signals, vehicle displays, radio ads, and verbal communication from people inside and outside our vehicles. As discussed in Chapter 5, we selectively attend to some of these activators, and ignore others. Only a portion of the activators we perceive actually influences our behavior. Understanding the six principles discussed in this chapter can help you predict which ones will influence behavior change.

Obviously, we do not need more activators in our lives. We certainly do need *more effective* activators to promote safety and health. It would be far better to make a few safety activators more powerful than to add more activators to a system already overloaded with information. We need to plan our safety activators carefully so the right safety directives receive the attention and ultimate action they deserve.

If you want an activator to motivate action, you need to imply consequences. The most powerful activators make the observer aware of consequences available following the performance of a target behavior. Consequences can be positive or negative, intrinsic or extrinsic to the task, and internal or external to the person. The next chapter explains the preceding sentence, which is key to getting the most beneficial behavior from an intervention process.

chapter eleven

Intervening with consequences

Consequences motivate behavior and related attitudes. This happens in various ways. Consequences can be positive or negative, intrinsic (natural) or extrinsic (extra) to a task, and internal or external to a person. These characteristics need to be considered when designing and evaluating intervention programs. This chapter explains why and provides principles and practical procedures for motivating people to work safely over the long term. In other words, I show you how to influence behavior and attitudes so that both are consistent with a Total Safety Culture.

"Every act you have ever performed since the day you were born was performed because you wanted something." — Dale Carnegie

The introductory quotation from Carnegie's classic book, *How to Win Friends and Influence People*, first published in 1936, represents a key principle of human motivation and behavior-based safety. Although supported by substantial research (Skinner, 1938), it actually runs counter to common sense.

Think about it. When people ask us why we did something, we are apt to say, "I wanted to do it," or "I was told to do it," or "I needed to do it." These explanations sound as if the cause of our behavior comes before we act. This perspective is supported by numerous pop psychology self-help books and audiotapes that say people motivate themselves with positive self-affirmations or optimistic thinking and enthusiastic intentions. In other words, behavior is caused by some external request, order, or signal or by an internal force, drive, desire, or need.

This chapter will explain the fallacy in this common sense and show ways to maximize the impact of an extrinsic reward process. Again, the research-supported principle is that activators *direct* behavior and consequences *motivate* behavior, but the type of consequence certainly influences the amount of motivation, as this chapter explains.

The power of consequences

Popular author and humorist Robert Fulghum (1988) wrote *All I Really Need to Know I Learned in Kindergarten,* claiming he learned all the basic rules or norms for socially acceptable adult behavior as a young child. The list of rules in Figure 11.1 was excerpted from Fulghum's famous book. Rules like *share everything, play fair, don't fight,*

❑ Share everything

❑ Play fair

❑ Don't hit others

❑ Put things back where you found them

❑ Clean up your own mess

❑ Don't take things that aren't yours

❑ Say you're sorry when you hurt someone

❑ Wash your hands before you eat

❑ Flush

❑ When you go out into the world, watch out for traffic, hold hands, and stick together

❑ And remember the Dick-and-Jane books and the first word you learned--the biggest word of all: **LOOK**

Figure 11.1 Basic rules of social life we learned well as children we do not necessarily follow as adults. Excerpted from Fulghum (1988).

and *clean-up your own mess* were taught to most of us early on. These are clearly ideal edicts to live by. Perhaps you still recall a teacher or parent using these rules to try to shape your behavior. Did it work? Do you follow each of these basic norms regularly, for no other reason or consequence except your realization that it's the right thing to do?

Imagine what a better world we would live in if everyone followed the simple rules listed in Figure 11.1 from a self-directed, principle-focused perspective. Alas, there are signs everywhere that this is not so.

The last two kindergarten rules in Figure 11.1 are directly relevant to safety and, in fact, reflect basic themes of this text. As discussed previously, safety needs people to stick together in a spirit of shared belonging and interdependence. However, sometimes we need activators to remind us of this critical rule and consequences to keep us working together for safety.

"LOOK," Fulghum's last rule, is key to behavior-based safety and to achieving a Total Safety Culture. This implies the "defensive working style" employees need to adopt. In a Total Safety Culture, everyone looks for ways to improve safety by intervening to reduce at-risk behaviors and increase safe behaviors. In Chapter 10, we discussed ways to intervene with activators. Here, we focus on the more powerful intervention approach — manipulating consequences.

Intrinsic vs. extrinsic consequences

Most applied behavioral scientists view "intrinsic motivation" differently from the description used in pop psychology books. The behavior-based perspective is

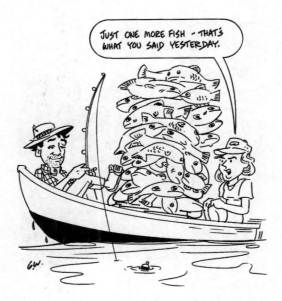

Figure 11.2 Some tasks are naturally motivating because of intrinsic consequences.

supported by research and our everyday experience. Plus, it's objective, practical, and useful for developing situations and programs to motivate behavior change.

Simply put, "intrinsic" does not mean "inside" people, where it cannot be observed, measured, and directly influenced. Rather, "intrinsic" refers to the nature of the task in which an individual is engaged. Intrinsically motivated tasks, or behaviors, lead *naturally* to external consequences that support the behavior (rewarding feedback) or give information useful for improving the behavior (corrective feedback).

Most athletic performance, for example, includes natural or intrinsic consequences that give rewarding or correcting feedback. These consequences, intrinsic to the task, tell us immediately how well we have performed at swinging a golf club, shooting a basketball, or casting a fishing lure, for example. They motivate us to keep trying, sometimes after adjusting our behavior as a result of the natural feedback directly related, or intrinsic, to the task.

Take a look at the fisherman in Figure 11.2. Some psychologists would claim he's motivated from within, or self-motivated. They use the term "intrinsic motivation" to refer to this state. In contrast, the behavioral scientist points to the external consequences naturally motivating the fisherman's behavior. These cause him to focus so completely on the task at hand that he is not aware of his wife's mounting anger — or he is ignoring her. He may also be unaware that his supply of fish is creating a potential hazard. In a similar way, safety can be compromised because of excessive motivation for production. Rewards intrinsic to production can cause this motivation.

Notice that the "worker" in this picture does not receive a reward for every cast. In fact, he's on an intermittent reinforcement schedule. He catches a fish once in a while. This kind of reward schedule is most powerful in maintaining continuous behavior. Anyone who has gambled understands. Some say gambling is a disease, when in fact gambling is behavior maintained by intermittent rewarding consequences.

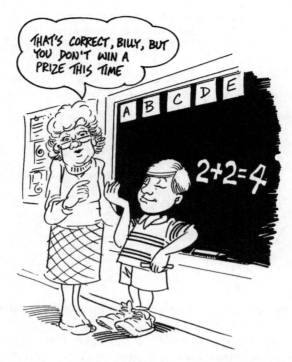

Figure 11.3 External rewards can reduce internal motivation.

Some tasks do not provide intrinsic or natural feedback. In this case, it's necessary to add an extrinsic, or extra consequence to support or redirect the behavior. Many, if not most, safety behaviors fall in this category.

In fact, many safety practices have intrinsic negative consequences, such as discomfort, inconvenience, and reduced pace, that naturally discourage their occurrence. Thus, there's often a need for extrinsic supportive consequences, like intermittent praise, recognition, novelties, and credits redeemable for prizes, to shape and maintain safe behaviors. The intent is not to control people, but to help people control their own behavior by offering positive reasons for making the safe choice.

Now look at the student in Figure 11.3. He expects an extrinsic positive consequence for completing an accurate calculation. Do you see a problem here? Sure, the pupil should feel good about deriving the right answer. In other words, the intrinsic consequence of completing a task correctly should be perceived as valuable and rewarding by the student. The student should perceive the important payoff as getting the right answer.

Now we are talking about a person's interpretation of the situation, which I refer to as "internal" consequences in the next section. First, let's understand a very important point reflected in Figure 11.3. Whenever there is an observable intrinsic consequence to a task, the instructor, supervisor, or safety coach needs to help the performer see that consequence and realize its importance. In other words, we need to help people perceive the intrinsic consequences of their performance and show appreciation and pride in that outcome. This helps to make the intrinsic consequence rewarding to the performer, thereby facilitating ongoing motivation.

So, if the teacher in Figure 11.3 displayed genuine approval and delight in the student's achievement, another extrinsic reward might not be needed to keep the performer motivated.

Internal vs. external consequences

The intrinsic and extrinsic consequences discussed so far are external to the individual. In other words, they can be observed by another person. Behavioral scientists focus on these types of consequences because they can be objective and scientific when dealing with external, observable aspects of people.

Behavioral scientists, however, do not deny the existence of internal factors that motivate action. There is no doubt that we talk to ourselves before and after our behaviors, and this self-talk influences our performance. We often give ourselves internal verbal instructions, called intentions, before performing certain behaviors. After our activities, we often evaluate our performance with internal consequences. In the process, we might motivate ourselves to press on (with self-commendation) or to stop (with self-condemnation).

When it comes to safety and health, internal consequences to support the right behavior are terribly important. Remember, external and intrinsic (natural) consequences for safe behaviors are not readily available, and we cannot expect to receive sufficient support (extra consequences) from others to sustain our proactive, safe, and healthy choices. So we need to talk to ourselves with sincere conviction to boost our intentions. To keep ourselves going, we also need to give ourselves genuine self-reinforcement after we do the right thing. When we receive special external consequences from others for our efforts, we need to savor these and use them later to bolster our self-reinforcement.

Managing consequences for safety

At this point, I'm sure you appreciate the special message reflected in Figure 11.4. Submitting safety suggestions is an activity not typically followed by external motivating consequences. In many work cultures, the idea of safety suggestions has long since passed. The suggestion boxes are empty. Does this mean there are no more good suggestions? Is the work force not creative enough? You know the answer to both of these questions is a resounding "no."

Let me give you an example. I once worked with safety leaders at a Toyota Motor manufacturing plant in Georgetown, KY, whose 6,000 employees submitted more than 35,000 quality, production, or safety-related suggestions in 1994. A greater number of suggestions were expected in 1995. Many employees in this culture are motivated internally to submit suggestions, but external consequences are in place to keep the process going.

Employees receive timely feedback regarding the utility and feasibility of every suggestion, and if the suggestion is approved, they are empowered to implement it themselves. Also, the individual or team responsible receives ten percent of the savings for the first year that result from the implemented suggestion. Such external, extra and meaningful — in this case economic — consequences motivate a large work force to make a difference.

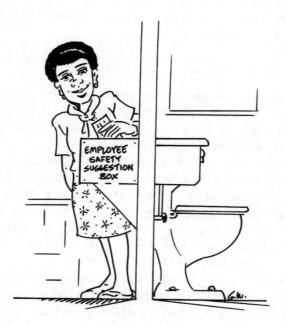

Figure 11.4 Some tasks require supportive consequences.

The case against negative consequences

To remove influences supporting at-risk behavior, it's often tempting to use a punishment or penalty. All that's needed is a policy statement or some type of top-down mandate specifying a soon, certain, and sizable negative consequence following specific observable risky behaviors. Could this contingency be powerful enough not to override the many natural positive consequences for taking risks?

Yes, behavioral scientists have found negative consequences can permanently suppress behavior if the punishment is severe, certain, and immediate. However, before using "the stick," you should understand the practical limitations and undesirable side effects of using negative consequences to influence behavior.

Escape. Animals and people attempt to avoid situations with a predominance of negative consequences. Sometimes, this means staying away from those who administer the punishment. Humans will often attempt to escape from negative consequences by simply "tuning out" or perhaps cheating or lying. Of course the ultimate escape from excessive negative consequences is suicide. Indeed, it is not uncommon for an individual to commit suicide in order to escape control by aversive stimulation, which can include the intractable pain of an incurable disease, physical or psychological abuse from a family member, or perceived harassment by an employee or coworker.

Unpleasant attitudes or emotional feelings are produced when people work to escape or avoid negative consequences. As shown in Figure 11.5, negative consequences can influence behavior dramatically, but such situations are usually unpleasant for the "victim." Under fear arousal conditions, people will be motivated to do the right thing, but only when they have to. They feel controlled, and as discussed

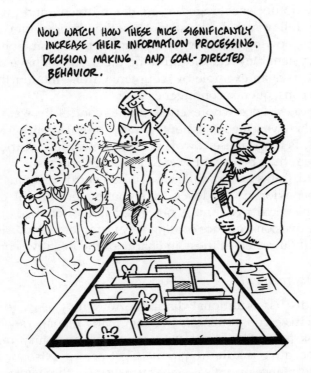

Figure 11.5 Fear of negative consequences is motivating.

in Chapter 6, this can lead to distress and burnout. Obviously, this type of contingency and side effect is incompatible with a Total Safety Culture where people feel "in control" and are ready and willing to go beyond the call of duty for another person's safety and health.

Aggression. Instead of escaping, people might choose to attack those perceived to be in charge. For example, murder in the workplace is rapidly increasing in the United States, and the most frequent cause appears to be reaction to or frustration with control by negative means. Aggressive reaction to this kind of control, however, might not be directed at the source.

An employee frustrated by top-down aversive control at work might not assault his boss directly, but rather slow down production, sabotage a safety program, steal supplies, or vandalize industrial property. Or the employee might react with spousal abuse. Then the abused spouse might react by slapping a child. The child, in turn, might punch a younger sibling and the younger sibling might punch a hole in a wall or kick the family pet — all as a result of perceived control by negative consequences.

Apathy. Apathy is a generalized suppression of behavior. In other words, the negative consequences not only suppress the target behavior but might also inhibit the occurrence of desirable behaviors. Regarding safety, this could mean a decrease in employee involvement. When people feel controlled by negative consequences, they are apt to simply resign themselves to doing only what is required. Going beyond the call of duty for a coworker's health or safety is out of the question.

Countercontrol. No one likes feeling controlled; situations that influence these feelings in people do not encourage buy-in, commitment, and involvement. In fact, some people only follow top-down rules when they believe they can get caught, as typified by drivers slowing down when noticing a police car. Some people look for ways to beat the system they feel is controlling them, so you have drivers purchasing radar detectors. This is an example of "countercontrol," the fourth undesirable side effect of negative consequence contingencies.

I met an employee once who exerted countercontrol by wearing safety glasses without lenses. When wearing his "safety frames," he got attention and approval from certain coworkers. Perhaps these coworkers were rewarded vicariously when seeing him beat the system they perceived was controlling them also.

Figure 11.6 illustrates an example of countercontrol. Although the supervisors might view the behavior as "feedback," it's countercontrol if it occurred to regain control or assert personal freedom. A perceived loss of control or freedom is most likely when a negative consequence contingency is implemented. Also, countercontrol behavior is typically directed at those in charge of the negative consequences.

Discipline and involvement

Let's specifically discuss traditional discipline for safety — a form of top-down control with negative consequences. I've met many managers who include a "discipline session" as part of the corrective action for an injury report. The injured employee gets a negative lecture from a manager or supervisor whose safety record and personal performance appraisal were tarnished by the injury.

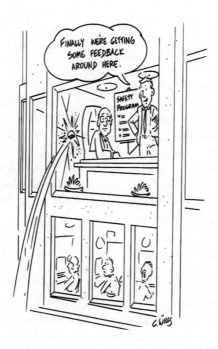

Figure 11.6 Countercontrol is usually directed at those in charge of negative consequences.

These "discipline sessions" are unpleasant for both parties and, certainly, do not encourage personal commitment or buy-in to the safety mission of the company. Instead, the criticized and embarrassed employees are simply reminded of the top-down control aspects of corporate safety, usually resulting in increased commitment *not* to volunteer for safety programs nor to encourage others to participate. In this case, the culture loses the involvement of invaluable safety participants.

What about progressive discipline? Whenever I teach behavior management principles and procedures, the question of how to deal with the repeat offender frequently comes up. Are there not times when punishment is necessary? Does not an individual who "willfully" breaks the rules after repeated warnings or confrontations deserve a penalty? Through progressive discipline these individuals receive top-down penalties, starting with verbal warning, then written warnings, and eventually dismissal. In some cases, dismissal is the best solution for noncooperative individuals who can be a divisive and dangerous factor in the workforce. Fortunately, this worst case scenario is rare.

The standard progressive discipline approach in safety enforcement includes three steps. After the third infraction, it's common to send the employee home for a certain number of days without pay. In other words, "three strikes and you're out." But the wrongdoer is not out for good. The individual is usually allowed back "in the game." Here's the critical question: Is the person a better "player" upon his or her return?

When employees are punished by being temporarily dismissed, we expect them to perform better when they return to work. In other words, we hope they learn something from this demeaning punishment. We also hope the learning is more than how to avoid getting caught next time.

Actually, whether the right or wrong kind of learning occurs in this situation depends on one key factor — attitude. If the employee is angry and does not own up to a calculated risk, useful learning is unlikely. If negative or hostile emotions develop in an employee as a result of the dismissal, don't expect the employee to return to work with a more pleasant and cooperative demeanor. Instead, expect a more disgruntled worker, who might give lip service to following the safety rules to avoid another dismissal but will likely share a negative attitude with anyone willing to listen. As we have all experienced, returning a "rotten apple" to a barrel makes other apples it contacts rotten also.

Positive discipline. One way to avoid this problem is not to send an employee home *without pay*. Instead, dismiss the employee *with pay*. Grote (1995) calls this "positive discipline." This is not about docking wages for a safety infraction. It's about finding a meaningful way to reduce a behavioral discrepancy. Now, this is not a free vacation day by any stretch of the imagination. The employee is required to think about the calculated risk and decide what can be done to eliminate such at-risk behavior. By not withholding wages, this evaluative process is not tainted by a negative or hostile attitude.

It should be clear that one option for the employee to consider is not to return to work. The individual should seriously consider whether he or she can meet the safety standards of the company. Is it too difficult to perform consistently with the paradigm of safety as a core value?

It's unlikely a person will admit to not holding safety as a core value. Thus, it's realistic and relevant for the employee to conduct a behavioral analysis (as outlined in Chapter 9), and then develop a personal corrective action plan for reducing the behavioral discrepancy implied by the rule infraction or calculated risk. Thus, at the end of the dismissal day(s), the ultimate deliverable is a specific list of things the employee will do to reduce the behavioral discrepancy and realign work practice with safety as a value.

This corrective action plan should include a specification of environmental and interpersonal supports the individual will summon in order to meet an improvement objective. For example, the employee might recommend a modification of a workstation to make the desired behavior more convenient or add an activator to the area as a behavioral reminder. The action plan might also include a solicitation of social support by requesting certain coworkers offer directive and/or supportive feedback (as detailed in Chapter 12).

It's critical for a supervisor or safety leader to review this corrective action plan as soon as the employee returns to work. Both parties must agree that the plan is reasonable, feasible, and cost effective. It's likely mutual agreement and commitment to a suitable action plan will require significant discussion, consensus building, and refinement of the document. The final document of the plan should be signed by both parties. When a person signs a commitment that took some effort to develop, the probability of compliance is greatly enhanced.

"Dos" and "don'ts" of safety rewards

Now let's look at the flip side of discipline — rewards. In one-on-one situations with children at home or in school, using positive consequences to increase desirable behavior is straightforward and easy. However, using rewarding consequences effectively with adults in work settings is easier said than done, especially when it comes to safety. Throughout my 35 years of professional experience in motivational psychology, I have seen more inappropriate reward programs in occupational safety than in any other area. This is unfortunate because the effective use of extra positive consequences is often critically important to overcoming the readily available influences supporting risky behavior.

Doing it wrong

Most incentive/reward programs for occupational safety do not specify behavior. Employees are rewarded for avoiding a work injury or for achieving a certain number of "safe work days." So, what behavior is motivated? Not to report injuries.

If having an injury loses one's reward, or worse, the reward for an entire work group, there's pressure to avoid reporting that injury, if possible. Many of these nonbehavioral, outcome-based incentive programs involve substantial peer pressure because they use a group-based contingency. That is, if anyone in the company or work group is injured, everyone loses the reward. Not surprisingly, I've seen coworkers cover for an injured employee in order to keep accumulating "safe days" and not lose their chance at a reward possibility.

These incentive programs might decrease the numbers of reported injuries, at least over the short term, but corporate safety is obviously not improved. Indeed, such programs often create apathy or helplessness regarding safety achievement. Employees develop the perspective that they cannot really control their injury record, but must cheat or beat the system to celebrate the "achievement" of an injury reduction goal.

Doing it right

Here are seven basic guidelines for establishing an effective incentive/reward program to motivate the occurrence of safety-related behaviors and improve industrial health and safety:

1. The behaviors required to achieve a safety reward should be specified and perceived as achievable by all participants.
2. Everyone who meets the behavioral criteria should be rewarded.
3. It's better for many participants to receive small rewards than for one person to receive a big reward.
4. The rewards should be displayed and represent safety achievement. Coffee mugs, hats, shirts, sweaters, blankets, or jackets with a safety message are preferable to rewards that will be hidden, used, or spent.
5. Contests should not reward one group at the expense of another.
6. Groups should not be penalized or lose their rewards for failure by an individual.
7. Progress toward achieving a safety reward should be systematically monitored and publicly posted for all participants.

Guideline 2 recommends against the popular lottery or raffle drawing. As illustrated in Figure 11.7, a lottery results in one "lucky" winner being selected and a large number of "unlucky" losers. The announcement of a raffle drawing might get many people excited, and if lottery tickets are dispensed for specific safe behaviors, there

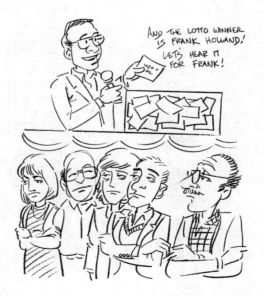

Figure 11.7 Raffle drawings that result in few "lucky" winners and many "unlucky" losers can do more harm than good.

is some motivational benefit. Eventually, however, the valuable reward is received by a lucky few. Also, I perceive a disadvantage in linking chance with safety. It's bad enough we use the word "accident" in the context of safety processes, as I pointed out in Chapter 3.

I've worked with a number of safety directors who used a lottery incentive program and vowed they'd never do it again. The big raffle prize, such as a snow-mobile, pick-up truck, or television set, is displayed in a prominent location. Everyone gets excited — temporarily — about the possibility of winning. Their attention is directed, however, at the big prize instead of the real purpose of the program: to keep everyone safe. *The material reward in an incentive program should not be perceived as the major payoff.* Incentives are only reminders to do the right thing, and rewards serve as feedback and a statement of appreciation for doing the right thing.

More important than external rewards is the way they are delivered. Rewards should not be perceived as a means of controlling behavior but as a declaration of sincere gratitude for making a contribution. If many people receive this recognition, you have many deposits in the emotional bank accounts of potential actively caring participants. That's why it's better to reward many than few (Guideline 3).

When rewards include a safety logo or message (Guideline 4), they become acti-vators for safety when displayed as illustrated in Figure 11.8. Also, if the safety message or logo was designed by representatives from the target population, the reward takes on special meaning (as discussed in Chapter 10). Special items like these cannot be purchased anywhere and, from the perspective of internal consequences, they are more valuable than money.

As portrayed in Figure 11.9, contests that pit one group against another can lead to an undesirable win–lose situation (Guideline 5). Safety needs to be perceived as win–win. This means developing a contract of sorts with each employee that makes

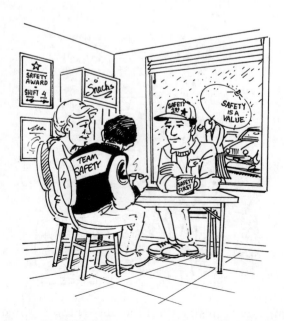

Figure 11.8 Rewards with safety messages are special to those who earn them.

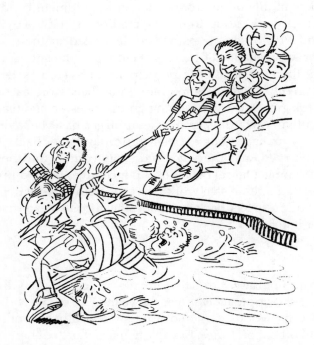

Figure 11.9 Safety contests can motivate unhealthy competition.

everyone a stockholder in achieving a Total Safety Culture. Everyone in the organization is on the same team. Team performance within departments or work groups can be motivated by providing team rewards or bonuses for team achievement. Every team that meets the "bonus" criteria should be eligible for the reward. In other words, Guideline 2 should be applied when developing incentive/reward programs to motivate team performance.

Obviously, developing and administering an effective incentive/reward program for safety requires a lot of dedicated effort. There is no quick fix, but it's worth doing, if you take the time to do it right. As Aubrey Daniels wisely stated, "If you think this is easy, you're doing it wrong" (2000, page 179). Let's examine an exemplary case study.

An exemplary incentive/reward program

In 1992, I consulted with the safety steering committee of a Hoechst Celanese company of about 2000 employees to develop a plant-wide incentive program that followed each of the guidelines given previously. The steering committee, including four hourly and four salary employees, met several times to identify specific behavior-consequence contingencies. That is, they needed to decide what behaviors should earn what rewards. Their plan was essentially a "credit economy" where certain safe behaviors, which could be achieved by all employees, earned certain numbers of "credits."

At the end of the year, participants exchanged their credits for a choice of different prizes, all containing a special safety logo. The variety of behaviors earning credits included attending monthly safety meetings; special participation in safety meetings; leading a safety meeting; writing, reviewing, and revising a job safety analysis; and conducting periodic audits of environmental and equipment conditions and certain work practices. For a work group to receive credits for audit activities, the results of environmental and PPE observations had to be posted in the relevant work areas. Only one behavior was penalized by a loss of credits — the late reporting of an injury.

At the start of the new year, each participant received a "safety credit card" for tallying ongoing credit earnings. Some individual behaviors earned credits for the person's entire work group, thus promoting group cohesion and teamwork. The audit aspect of this incentive/reward program exemplifies a basic behavior-based principle for health and safety management — observation and feedback. Employees were systematically observed, and they received soon, certain, and positive feedback (a reward) after performing a target behavior. An incentive/reward program is only one of several methods to increase safe work practices with observation and feedback. In the next chapter, I address feedback more specifically as an external and extra consequence to prevent injuries.

Safety thank-you cards

I'd be remiss if I did not describe "safety thank-you cards" in a discussion of exemplary incentive/reward approaches. Over the years, I've seen a wide variety of thank-you cards designed by work teams and used successfully at a number of industrial sites, including Abbott Laboratories, Exxon Chemical, Ford, General Motors, Hercules, Hoechst Celanese, Kal Kan, Logan Aluminum, Phillip Morris, Westinghouse Hanford Company, and Weyerhaeuser.

At some locations, thank-you cards were used in a raffle drawing, exchangeable for food, drinks, or trinkets, or displayed on a plant bulletin board as a "safety honor roll." Sometimes the cards could be accumulated and exchanged for tee shirts, caps, or jackets with messages or logos signifying safety achievement. At several plants, the person who delivered a thank-you card returned a receipt naming the recognized employee and describing the behavior earning the consequence, thus creating objective information to define a "safe employee of the month."

At a few locations, the thank-you cards took on a special actively caring meaning. Specifically, when deposited in a special collection container, each thank-you card was worth 25¢ toward corporate contributions to a local charity or to needy families in the community. The actively caring card used at the Hoechst Celanese plant in Rock Hill, SC, is shown in Figure 11.10. The back of the card included a colorful peel-off symbol which the recognized employee could affix in any number of places as a personal reminder of the recognition. I was surprised but pleased to see a large number of these thank-you stickers on employees' hard hats. Obviously, this actively caring thank-you approach to safety recognition has great potential as an inexpensive but powerful tool for motivating safe behavior.

Motivational leverage with this simple actively caring thank-you card was illustrated a few years ago at the Hercules chemical plant in Portland, OR. The actively caring cards delivered for safety-related behaviors were similar to the one illustrated in Figure 11.10, except the peel-off sticker depicted the company logo — a rhinoceros. The incentive/reward contingency was simply stated: Give an actively caring thank-you card and "rhino sticker" to anyone who goes beyond the call of duty for safety or health.

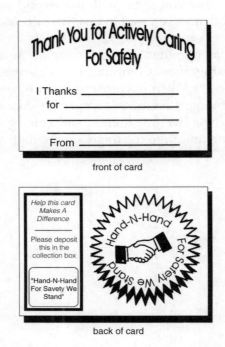

front of card

back of card

Figure 11.10 This Actively Caring Thank-You Card offers reward leverage.

Here is special motivational leverage. Every actively caring card received and then deposited in a designated "actively caring for others" box was worth $1.00 to purchase toys for disadvantaged children in and around Portland. With this program, the 64 line workers at this chemical plant contributed more than $1750 during the Christmas holidays of 1996. Guess who picked out and delivered the toys? Children of the employees. Now that's special actively caring leverage from a simple behavior-based incentive/reward program.

In conclusion

Writing this book was challenging, tedious, overwhelming, tiresome, sacrificing, and exhausting. Observers were apt to say I was self-directed and intrinsically motivated. Of course I know better, and so do you.

Incidentally, I literally wrote the various drafts of this text. I have never learned to type and, therefore, have never benefited from the technological magic of computer word processing. My colleagues explain that it's not necessary to be a skilled typist to reap the many intrinsic benefits of preparing a manuscript on a computer. "I type slowly with only one finger," some say, "and still enjoy the wonderful benefits of high-tech computer word processing. I could never go back to preparing a manuscript by hand. You don't know what you're missing."

I'm sure you noticed my disparate uses of "intrinsic" in the prior paragraphs and you now understand the two meanings of this popular motivational term. Are my friends and colleagues so enthusiastic about computer-based word processing because of intrinsic (internal) motivation or because of intrinsic (natural) consequences linked to their computer use? I hope you agree with the second reason. But, of course, the natural rewarding consequences can lead to positive self-talk and internal (unobservable) motivation.

Word processing on a computer allows for rapid "quick-fix" control of letters, words, sentences, and paragraphs. Computer users also can walk to a printer and obtain a typed, "hard copy" of their document for study, revision, or dissemination. All these soon, certain, and positive consequences are connected naturally to word-processing behavior. No wonder my friends and colleagues are motivated about computer word processing and urge me to get on the high-tech "band wagon."

chapter twelve

Intervening as a behavior-change agent

This chapter presents the principles and procedure of safety coaching — a key behavior-change process for safety improvement. The letters of COACH represent the critical sequential steps of safety coaching: Care, Observe, Analyze, Communicate, Help. This coaching process is clearly relevant for improving behaviors in areas other than safety and in settings other than the workplace. Behavior-based feedback is critical for improvement in everything we do. This chapter shows you how to give feedback effectively.

"There are risks and costs to a program of action. But they are far less than the long range risks and costs of comfortable inaction." — John F. Kennedy

Large-scale behavior change is impossible without intervention agents — people willing and able to step in on behalf of another person's safety. In a Total Safety Culture, everyone feels responsible for safety, pursuing it daily. They go beyond the call of duty to identify at-risk conditions and behaviors and intervene to correct them. This chapter is about becoming a behavior-focused change agent.

In simplest terms, this means observing and supporting safe behaviors or observing and correcting at-risk behaviors. It might involve designing and implementing a particular intervention process for a work team, organizational culture, or an entire community. Or it might mean merely engaging in behavior-focused communication between an observer (the intervention agent) and the person observed. This is safety coaching and, to be effective, certain principles and guidelines need to be followed.

Intervening as a safety coach

Coaching is essentially a process of one-on-one observation and feedback. The coach systematically observes the behaviors of another person and provides behavioral feedback on the basis of the observations. Safety coaches recognize and support the safe behaviors they observe and offer constructive feedback to reduce the occurrence of any at-risk behaviors. This chapter specifies the steps of safety coaching, points out trainable skills needed to accomplish the process, and illustrates tools and support mechanisms for increasing effectiveness.

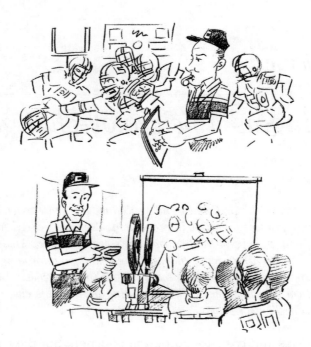

Figure 12.1　Systematic observation and feedback are key to effective coaching.

The term "coach" is very familiar to us in an athletic context. In fact, winning coaches practice the basic observation and feedback processes needed for effective safety coaching. They follow most of the guidelines reviewed here. As illustrated in Figure 12.1, the most effective team coaches observe the ongoing behaviors of individual players and record their observations in systematic fashion, using a team roster, behavioral checklist, or videotape.

Football coaches, for instance, spend hours and hours analyzing film. Then they deliver specific and constructive feedback to team members to instruct, support, or motivate desirable behavior and/or to decrease undesirable behavior. Sometimes the feedback is given in a group session, perhaps by critiquing videotapes of team competition. At other times, the feedback is given individually in a personal one-on-one conversation. Usually, the one-on-one format has greater impact on individual performance.

The five letters of the word COACH can be used to remember the basic ingredients of the most effective coaching — whether coaching the members of a winning athletic team or the individuals in a work group striving for an injury-free workplace. This is my favorite instructional acronym because it not only contains the components of an effective coaching process, but lists them in the sequence in which they should occur.

"C" for care

Caring is the basic underlying motivation for coaching. Safety coaches truly care about the health and safety of their coworkers and they act on such caring. In other words, they "actively care." When people realize by a safety coach's words and body language that he or she cares, they are more apt to listen to and accept the coach's advice. When people know you care, they care what you know.

Our emotional bank accounts. Stephen Covey (1989) explained the value of interdependence among people — exemplified by appropriate safety coaching — with the metaphor of an "emotional bank account." People develop an emotional bank account with others through personal interaction. Deposits are made when the holder of the account views a particular interaction to be positive, as when he or she feels recognized, appreciated, or listened to. Withdrawals from a person's emotional bank account occur whenever that individual feels criticized, humiliated, or less appreciated, usually as a result of personal interaction.

Sometimes, it's necessary to offer constructive criticism or even state extreme displeasure with another person's behavior. However, if such negative discourse occurs on an "overdrawn or bankrupt account," this corrective feedback will have limited impact. In fact, continued withdrawals from an overdrawn account can lead to defensive or countercontrol reactions. The person will simply ignore the communication or actually do things to discredit the source or undermine the process or system implicated in the communication.

Thus, safety coaches need to demonstrate a caring attitude throughout their personal interactions with others. This maintains healthy emotional bank accounts — operating in the "black." The woman in Figure 12.2 is requesting a deposit along with the withdrawal. Our emotional reaction to police officers depends on the proportion of deposits vs. withdrawals we have experienced with them.

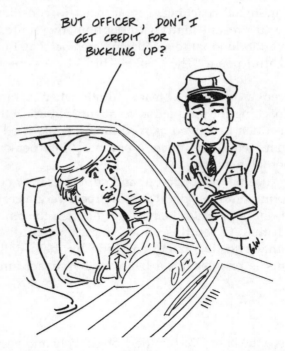

Figure 12.2 Our attitude toward police officers would be more positive if we received deposits along with withdrawals.

The Cookie Thief
By Valerie Cox

A woman was waiting at an airport one night, With several long hours before her flight. She hunted for a book in the airport shop, Bought a bag of cookies and found a place to drop.	He offered her half, as he ate the other. She snatched it from him and thought, "Oh, brother, This guy has some nerve and he's also rude, Why, he didn't even show any gratitude!"
She was engrossed in her book, but happened to see, That a man beside her, as bold as could be Grabbed a cookie or two from the bag between, Which she tried to ignore, to avoid a scene.	She had never known when she had been so galled And sighed with relief when her flight was called. She gathered her belongings and headed for the gate, Refusing to look back at the " thieving ingrate."
She read, munched cookies and watched the clock, As the gutsy "cookie thief" diminished her stock. She was getting more irritated as the minutes ticked by, Thinking, "If I wasn't so nice, I'd blacken his eye!"	She boarded the plane and sank in her seat, Then sought her book, which was almost complete. As she reached in her baggage, she gasped with surprise. There was her bag of cookies in front of her eyes!
With each cookie she took, he took one too. When only one was left, she wondered what he'd do. With a smile on his face and a nervous laugh, He took the last cookie and broke it in half.	"If mine are here" she moaned with despair, "Then the others were his and he tried to share!" Too late to apologize, she realized with grief, That she was the rude one, the ingrate, the thief!

Figure 12.3 Independence from one person can stifle interdependence from another.

A shared responsibility. People are often unwilling to coach or to be coached for safety because they view safety from an individualistic perspective. To them, it's a matter of individual or personal responsibility. This is illustrated by the verbal expression or internal script, "If Molly and Mike want to put themselves at risk, that's their problem, not mine." For some people a change in personal attitude or perspective is needed in order to motivate coaching. People need to consider safety coaching a shared responsibility to prevent injuries throughout the entire work culture. This requires a shift from an individual to a collective perspective. But this is not easy, as reflected in the insightful poem "The Cookie Thief" by Valerie Cox, reproduced in Figure 12.3.

Many people accept a collective or team attitude when it comes to work productivity and quality. Coaching for production or quality is part of the job, but coaching for personal safety is often perceived as meddling. People need to understand that safety-related behaviors require as much, if not more, interpersonal observation and feedback as any other job activity.

One way to convince people to accept and support safety coaching as a shared responsibility is to point out their plant's injury record for a certain period of time. While an injury did not happen to them, it did happen to someone, and everyone certainly cares about that. Given this underlying caring attitude, the challenge is to convince others that effective safety coaching by them will reduce injuries to their coworkers. This is enabled by a behavior-based accountability system, as discussed next.

"O" for observe

Safety coaches observe the behavior of others objectively and systematically, with an eye for supporting safe behavior and correcting at-risk behavior. Behavior that illustrates going beyond "the call of duty" for the safety of another person should be

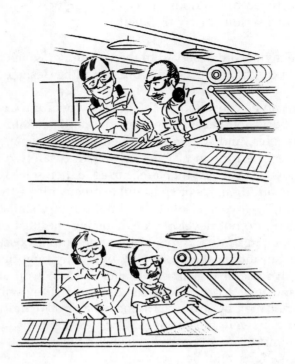

Figure 12.4 Safety coaches are up-front about their intentions and
ask permission before observing.

especially supported. This is the sort of behavior that contributes significantly to safety
improvement and can be increased through rewarding feedback. As illustrated in
Figure 12.4, a safety observer does not hide or spy, and always asks permission first.
Only with permission should an observation process proceed.

Observing behavior for supportive and constructive feedback is easy if the coach:

1. Knows exactly what behaviors are desired and undesired (an obvious requirement for athletic coaching)
2. Takes the time to observe occurrences of these behaviors in the work setting

It's often advantageous — and usually essential — to develop a checklist of
safe and at-risk behaviors and to rank them in terms of risk. Ownership and
commitment are increased when workers develop their own behavioral checklists.

Developing a critical behavioral checklist. Observation checklists can be generic
or job-specific. A generic checklist is used to observe behaviors that may occur during
several jobs. A job-specific checklist is designed for one particular job. Deciding which
items to include on a critical behavior checklist (CBC) is a very important part of the
coaching process. A CBC enables coaches to look for critical behaviors. A critical
behavior is a behavior that:

1. Has led to a large number of injuries or near hits in the past
2. Could potentially contribute to a large number of injuries or near hits because
   many people perform the behavior

3. Has previously led to a serious injury or a fatality
4. Could lead to a serious injury or fatality

If only a few behaviors are observed in the beginning, which is often a good way to start a large-scale coaching process, a CBC should be designed for only the most critical behaviors.

Several sources can be consulted to obtain behaviors for a CBC, including injury records, near-hit reports, job hazard analyses, standard operating procedures, rules and procedural manuals, and the workers themselves. People already know a lot about their own safety performance. They know which safety rules they sometimes ignore, and they know when a near hit has occurred to themselves or to others because of at-risk behavior. In addition, it's often useful to obtain advice from the plant doctor, nurse, safety director, or anyone else who maintains injury statistics for the plant.

When starting out, do not develop an exhaustive checklist of critical behaviors. A list can get quite long in a hurry. A long list for one-on-one observations can appear overwhelming and can inhibit the process. As with anything that's new and needs voluntary support, it's useful to start small and build. With practice, people find a CBC easy to use, and they accept additions to the list. They will also contribute in valuable ways to refine the CBC, from clarifying behavioral definitions to recommending behavioral additions and substitutions. The development and use of a CBC is really a continuous improvement process. Further development and refinement benefits coaching observations, and vice versa.

A work group on a mission to develop a CBC needs to meet periodically to select critical behaviors to observe. I have found the worksheet depicted in Figure 12.5 useful in beginning the development of a CBC. Through interactive discussions, work groups define safe and at-risk behaviors in their own work areas relevant to each category. The category on body positioning and protecting, for example, includes specific ways workers should protect themselves from environment or equipment hazards. This can range from using certain personal protective equipment to positioning their body parts in certain ways to avoid possible injury.

Some categories in Figure 12.5 may be irrelevant for certain work groups, like locking or tagging out equipment or complying with certain permit policies. A work group might add another general procedural category to cover particular work behaviors. Notice that defining safe and at-risk behaviors results in safety training in the best sense of the word. Participants learn exactly what safe behaviors are needed for a particular work process.

A list of work behaviors covering all the generic categories in Figure 12.5 can be extensive and overwhelming. This gives numerous opportunities for coaching feedback, but, remember, it takes time and practice to observe behaviors reliably — and to get used to being observed while working. I have found it useful to start the observation procedure with a brief CBC of four or five behaviors, and then build on the list with practice, group discussion, and more practice.

Scheduling observation sessions. There's no best way to arrange for coaching observations. The process needs to fit the setting and work process. This can only happen if workers themselves decide on the frequency and duration of the observations and derive a method for scheduling the coaching sessions. I have seen the protocol for effective coaching observations vary widely across plants, and across

Operating Procedures	Safe Observation	At-Risk Observation
BODY POSITIONING/PROTECTING *Positioning/protecting body parts* *(e.g., avoiding line of fire, using PPE,* *equipment guards, barricades, etc.).*		
VISUAL FOCUSING *Eyes and attention devoted to ongoing* *task(s).*		
COMMUNICATING *Verbal or nonverbal interaction that* *affects safety.*		
PACING OF WORK *Rate of ongoing work (e.g., spacing* *breaks appropriately, rushing).*		
MOVING OBJECTS *Body mechanics while lifting,* *pushing/pulling.*		
COMPLYING WITH LOCKOUT/TAGOUT *Following procedures for* *lockout/tagout*		
COMPLYING WITH PERMITS *Obtaining, then complying with* *permit(s). (e.g., confined space entry,* *hot work, excavation, open line, hot* *tap, etc.).*		

Figure 12.5 Use this worksheet to develop a generic critical behavior checklist (CBC).

departments within the same plant. The success of those processes has not varied predictably as a function of protocol.

The 350 employees at one Exxon Chemical plant, for example, designed a process calling for people to schedule their own coaching sessions with any two other employees. On days and at times selected by the person to be observed, two observers show up at the individual's worksite and use a CBC to conduct a systematic, 30-minute observation session. This plant started with only one scheduled observation per month, and observers were selected from a list of volunteers who had received special coaching training. One year later, employees scheduled two observations per month, and any plant employee could be called on to coach. With slight periodic revisions, this interpersonal coaching process has been in place for eight years (at the time of this writing) and it has enabled this plant to reach and sustain a record-low injury rate.

The Exxon procedure is markedly different from the "planned 60-second actively caring review" implemented at a Hoechst Celanese plant. For this one-on-one coaching process, all employees attempt to complete a one-minute observation of another employee's work practices in five general categories: body position, personal apparel, housekeeping, tools/equipment, and operating procedures. The initial plant goal was for each of the 800 employees to complete one 60-second behavioral observation every day. Results were entered into a computer file for a behavioral safety analysis of the work culture.

The CBC used for the one-minute coaching observations is shown in Figure 12.6. The front of each card includes the five behavioral categories, a column to check "safe"

Observer: _____	Location: _____	Date: _____		
Audit Category	Safe	At Risk	Feedback Targets: Safe	At Risk
Position				
Safe Apparel				
Housekeeeping				
Tools/Equip.				
Procedures				
Total				

Front of One-Minute Audit Card

Observation Targets	Safe	At Risk	Observation Targets	Safe	At -Risk

Position
  * Line of Fire
  * Falling
  * Pinch Points
  * Lifting
			Tools/Equip.
			  * Condition
			  * Use
			  * Guards		

Safe Apparel
  * Hair
  * Clothes
  * Jewelry
  * PPE
			Procedures
			  * SOPs
			  * JSAs
			  * Permits
			  * Lockout
			  * Barricade
			  * Equipment
			     Release		

Housekeeping
  * Floor
  * Equipment
  * Storage of
    Materials					

Back of One-Minute Audit Card

Figure 12.6 Employees used this critical behavior checklist for one-minute observations.

or "at risk" per category, and columns (feedback targets) to write comments about the observations. These comments facilitate a feedback session following the observation session, if it's convenient. The back of this CBC includes examples (memory joggers) related to each behavioral category on the front of the card. These examples summarize the category definitions developed by the CBC steering committee and determine whether "safe" or "at-risk" should be checked on the front of the card.

Critical features of the observation process. Duration, frequency, and scheduling procedures of CBC observations vary widely. Still, there are a few common features. First and foremost, the observer must ask permission before beginning an observation process. The name of the person observed must never be recorded. To build trust and increase participation, a "no" to a request to observe must be honored.

Asking permission to observe serves notice to work safely and, thus, biases the observation data, right? In other words, when workers give permission to be coached, their attention to safety will likely increase and they will try to follow all safety procedures. It's possible, though, for people to overlook safety precautions, even when trying their best. They could be unconsciously at risk. When people give permission to be coached, their willingness to accept and appreciate feedback is maximized, even when it's corrective.

What if people sneak around and conduct behavioral observations with no warning? This is in fact an unbiased plant-wide audit of work practices. It might even be accepted if those observed were not identified. However, if one-on-one coaching is added to this procedure, an atmosphere of mistrust can develop.

Safety coaching should not be a way to enforce rules or play "gotcha." It needs to be seen as a process to help people develop safe work habits through supportive and constructive feedback. Giving corrective feedback after "catching" an individual off-guard performing an at-risk behavior will likely lead to defensiveness and lack of appreciation, even for a well-intentioned effort. It can also reduce interpersonal trust and alienate a person toward the entire safety coaching process.

Feedback is essential. Each observation process with a CBC provides for tallying and graphing results as "percent safe behavior" on a group feedback chart. All checks for safe observations can be added and divided by the total number of checks (safe plus at-risk behaviors). The result is multiplied by 100 to yield percent safe behavior.

Applying this formula to checks written on the front of the CBC shown in Figure 12.6 results in a conservative estimate of percent safe behavior. That is because a safe check mark on the CBC in this application means that each separate behavior of a certain category is marked safe on the back. Thus, this calculation requires all behaviors relating to a particular observation category to be safe for a "safe" designation. A calculation based on individual behaviors rather than on an "all-or-none" classification of a "safe" or "at-risk" category generally results in higher percentages.

There's no best way to do these calculations. What's important is for participants to understand the meaning of the feedback percentages. As shown in the lower half of Figure 12.7, these percentages can be readily displayed on a group feedback chart or graph. While feedback percentages are valuable, it's vital to realize that the process is more important than the numbers.

The true value of the coaching process is not in the behavioral data, which are no doubt biased by uncontrollable factors, but in the behavior-based interaction between employees. I have actually seen observers get so caught up in recording the numbers, such as frequency of safe and at-risk behaviors, that they let coworkers continue to perform an at-risk behavior while they observe and check columns on a CBC.

An individual's safety must come before the numbers in any observation process. When observers see an at-risk behavior that immediately threatens a person's health or safety, they should intervene at once. They can usually pick up the observation process afterwards. On the other hand, if the CBC was partially completed before they stepped in, it might be most convenient to communicate other observations, especially if there are some safe behaviors to report. This "deposit" will help compensate for the "withdrawal" that was probably implicated by the need to stop a risky behavior.

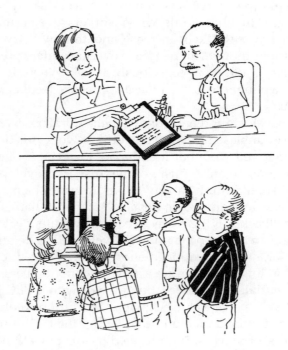

Figure 12.7 Feedback from a critical behavior checklist can be given
one-on-one and in groups.

"A" for analyze

When interpreting observations, safety coaches draw on their understanding of the ABC contingency (for activator–behavior–consequence) introduced in Chapter 8 and the behavior analysis principles discussed in Chapter 9. They realize observable reasons usually exist for why safe or risky behaviors occur They know certain dangerous behaviors are triggered by activators such as work demands, risky example setting by peers, and inconsistent messages from management. They also appreciate the fact that at-risk behaviors are often motivated by one or more natural consequences, including comfort, convenience, work breaks, and approval from peers or work supervisors.

This understanding is critical if safety coaching is to be a "fact-finding" rather than "fault-finding" process. It also leads to an objective and constructive analysis of the situations observed. This is how people discover the reasons behind at-risk behaviors and then design interventions to decrease them.

An ABC analysis can be done before giving feedback to the person observed or during the one-on-one feedback process. Discussing the activators and consequences that possibly influenced certain work practices can lead to environment or system improvements for decreasing at-risk behavior:

- Was the behavior observed activated by a work demand or a desire to go on break or leave work early?
- Does the design of the equipment or environment, or the ergonomic design of the task, influence at-risk behavior?

- Is certain PPE uncomfortable or difficult to use?
- Are fellow workers or supervisors activating dangerous behavior by requesting or demanding an excessive work pace?
- Are certain people motivating at-risk behavior from others by giving rewarding consequences, like words of appreciation, for work done quickly at the expense of safety?

Answers to these and other questions are explored with the observee in the next phase of safety coaching — the heart of the process.

"C" for communicate

A good coach is a good communicator. This means being an active listener and persuasive speaker. Because none of us is born with these skills, communication training sessions that incorporate role-playing exercises can be invaluable in developing the confidence and competence needed to send and receive behavioral feedback. Such training should emphasize the need to separate behavior (actions) from person factors (attitudes and feelings). This enables corrective feedback without stepping on feelings.

People need to understand that anyone can be at risk without even realizing it, as in "unconscious incompetence," and performance can only improve with behavior-specific feedback. Once this fact is established, corrective feedback that is appropriately given will be appreciated, regardless of who is giving the feedback. Work status is not a factor.

The right delivery. I remember key aspects of effective verbal presentation with the "SOFTEN" acronym listed in Figure 12.8. First, it's important for the observer to initiate communication with a friendly smile and an open (flexible) perspective.

Smile
Open
Friendly
Territory
Energy
   Enthusiasm
      Eye Contact
Name

Figure 12.8 Principles of effective sending can be remembered with SOFTEN.

"Territory" reflects the need to respect the fact that you are encroaching upon another person's work area. You should ask the person where it would be appropriate and safe to talk. It's also important to maintain a proper physical distance during this interaction.

Standing too close or too far from another person can cause interference and discomfort. There are prominent cultural differences in interpersonal distance norms. In the United States, an area closer than 18 inches to another person — measured nose to nose — is considered an intimate distance, with 0 to 6 inches reserved for comforting, protesting, lovemaking, wrestling, and other full-contact behaviors. The far phase of the intimate zone (6 to 18 inches) is used by individuals who are on very close terms.

Safety coaches in the United States should most likely communicate at a "personal distance" (18 inches to 4 feet). According to research by Edward Hall (1966), the near phase of the personal distance (18 to 30 inches) is reserved for those who are familiar with one another and on good terms. The far phase of the personal zone (2.5 to 4 feet) is typically used for social interactions between friends and acquaintances. This is likely to be the most common interaction zone for a workplace coaching session. Some coaching communication might occur at the near phase (4 to 7 feet) of Hall's social distance, which is typical for unacquainted individuals interacting informally. These distance recommendations are not hard and fast rules of conduct but rather personal territory norms we need to consider.

The "E" of our acronym represents three important directives to remember when coaching — energy, enthusiasm, and eye contact. Your energy and enthusiasm can activate concern and caring on the part of the person you are communicating with. We all know that excited, committed coaches can make "true believers" out of the troops — and that indifferent or distracted coaches can have the opposite effect. Actually, as depicted in Figure 12.9, our body language speaks louder than words.

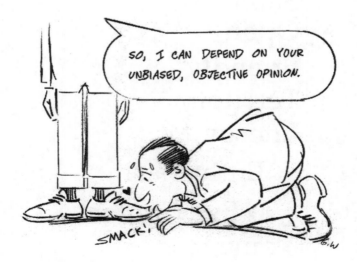

Figure 12.9 Body language communicates more than words.

Finally, we need to remember that the dearest word to anyone's ears is his or her own name. Refer to the other person by name, but make it clear the behavioral observations you have recorded will remain anonymous.

Individual feedback. Whether the aim is to support or correct, feedback should be specific and timely. It should specify a particular behavior and occur soon after the target behavior is performed. Also, it should be private, given one-on-one to avoid any interference or embarrassment from others. Corrective feedback is most effective if the alternative safe behavior is specified and potential solutions for eliminating the at-risk behavior are discussed.

Anyone giving feedback must actively listen to reactions. This is how a safety coach shows sincere concern for the feelings and self-esteem of the person on the receiving end of feedback. The best listeners give empathic attention with facial cues and posture, paraphrase to check understanding, prompt for more details, accept stated feelings without interpretation, and avoid arrogance such as "When I worked in your department, I always worked safely."

Figure 12.10 reviews the critical characteristics of effective rewarding and correcting feedback. This figure can be used as a guide for group practice sessions. Because it's not easy to give safety feedback properly and because many people feel awkward or uncomfortable doing it, practice is important.

Use Rewarding Feedback to Support Safe Behavior

- Give the feedback one-on-one and privately.
- Give the feedback as soon as possible after the observation process.
- Identify the safe behavior(s) observed.
- Be sincere and genuine.
- Express personal appreciation for setting the right example for others.

Use Correcting Feedback to Decrease At-Risk Behavior

- Give the feedback one-on-one and privately.
- Give the feedback as soon as possible after the observation process.
- Begin with acknowledgment of safe behavior(s) observed.
- Identify the at-risk behavior(s) observed.
- Specify the safe alternative to the at-risk behavior(s).
- Indicate concern for the person's welfare.
- Request commitment to avoid the at-risk behavior(s).

Figure 12.10 Maximize the beneficial impact of rewarding and correcting feedback with these key points.

"H" for help

The word "help" summarizes what safety coaching is all about. The purpose is to help an individual prevent injury by supporting safe work practices and correcting at-risk practices. It's critical, of course, that a coach's help is accepted. The four letters of HELP outline strategies to increase the probability that a coach's advice, directions, or feedback will be appreciated.

Humor. Safety is certainly a serious matter, but sometimes a little humor can add spice to our communications, increasing interest and acceptance. It can take the sting out of what some find to be an awkward situation. In fact, researchers have shown that laughter can reduce distress and even benefit our immune system.

Esteem. People who feel inadequate, unappreciated, or unimportant are not as likely to go beyond "the call of duty" to benefit the safety of themselves or others as people who feel capable and valuable (see Chapter 15 for support of this argument). The most effective coaches choose their words carefully, emphasizing the positive over the negative in order to build or avoid lessening another person's self-esteem. Although Figure 12.11 is humorous, it's unfortunately an accurate portrayal of the atmosphere in many organizational cultures, including the university environment in which I have worked for more than 30 years.

Listen. One of the most powerful and convenient ways to build self-esteem is to listen attentively to another person. This sends the signal that the listener cares about the person and his or her situation. And it builds self-esteem — "I must be valuable to the organization because my opinion is appreciated." After a safety coach listens actively, his or her message is more likely to be heard and accepted.

Praise. Praising others for their specific accomplishments is another powerful way to build self-esteem. If the praise targets a particular behavior, the probability of the

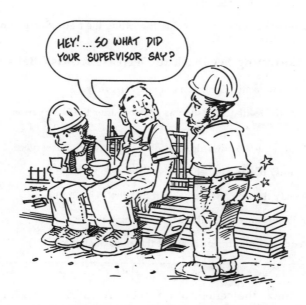

Figure 12.11   Standard feedback more often depreciates
than appreciates a person's self-esteem.

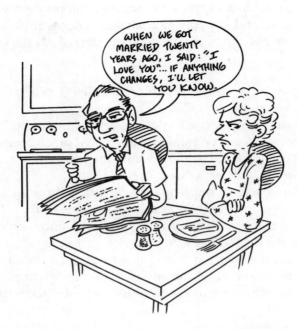

Figure 12.12 People need frequent rewarding feedback.

behavior reoccurring increases. This reflects the basic principle of positive reinforcement and motivates people to continue their safe work practices and look out for the safety of coworkers. Behavior-focused praising is a powerful rewarding consequence which not only increases the behavior it follows, but also increases a person's self-esteem. This, in turn, increases the individual's willingness to actively care for the safety of others, as I discuss more completely in Part 5 of this book.

Human nature directs more attention to mistakes than successes. Errors stick out and disrupt the flow, so they attract reaction and attempts to correct them. As illustrated in Figure 12.12, however, when things are going smoothly — and safely — there is usually no stimulus to signal success. A person's good performance is typically taken for granted. We need to resist the tendency to go with the flow, and sometimes express sincere appreciation for ongoing safe behavior. I give specifics on how to do this in the next chapter.

In conclusion

Safety coaching is a key intervention process for developing and maintaining a Total Safety Culture. In fact, the more employees effectively apply the principles of safety coaching discussed here, the closer an organization will come to achieving a Total Safety Culture. The same is true for preventing injury in the community and among our immediate family members at home. Indeed, we need to practice the principles of safety coaching in every situation where an injury could occur following at-risk behavior.

Systematic safety coaching throughout a work culture is certainly feasible in most settings. Large-scale success requires time and resources to develop materials, train necessary personnel, establish support mechanisms, monitor progress, and continually improve the process and support mechanisms whenever possible. For example, the following questions need to be answered at the start of developing an initial action plan:

- Who will develop the critical behavior checklist (CBC)?
- How extensive will the first CBC be?
- What information will be used to define critical behaviors?
- How will safety coaches be trained and receive practice and feedback?
- How many coaches will be trained initially and how can additional people volunteer to participate as a safety coach?
- How will the coaching sessions be scheduled, how often will people be coached, and how long will the coaching sessions last?
- Where will the group feedback graphs be posted, and who will be responsible for preparing the displays of safe behavior percentages?
- Who will be on the steering committee to oversee the safety coaching process, answer these and other questions about process implementation, maintain records, monitor progress, and refine procedural components whenever necessary?

This does not cover all the issues, yet the list might appear overwhelming at first. There is no formula for a quick-fix solution. Organizational cultures vary widely according to personnel, history, policy, the work process, environmental factors, and current contingencies. So implementation procedures need to be customized. There must be significant input from the people protected by the coaching process and from whom long-term participation is needed.

It's likely to take significant time, effort, and resources to achieve a plant-wide safety coaching process. With this end in mind, I recommend starting small to build confidence and optimism on small-win accomplishments. Then with patience and diligence, set long-term goals for continuous improvement. Remember to celebrate achievements that reflect successive approximations of your vision — an organization of people who consistently coach each other effectively to increase safe work practices and decrease at-risk behaviors.

chapter thirteen

Intervening with supportive conversation

Interpersonal conversation defines the culture in which we work. It can create conflict and build barriers to safety improvement or it can cultivate the kind of work culture needed to make a major breakthrough in injury prevention. Interpersonal conversation also affects our intrapersonal conversations or self-talk, which in turn influences our willingness to get involved in safety-improvement efforts. This chapter explains the reciprocal impact of inter- and intrapersonal conversation and offers guidelines for aligning both toward the achievement of a Total Safety Culture.

"Leadership is the ability to persuade others to do what you want them to do because they want to do it." — Dwight Eisenhower

This chapter is about interpersonal conversation and coaching, but unlike Chapter 12 on systematic safety coaching, the emphasis is on brief informal communication to support safe behaviors and help them become more fluent. How we talk with others (interpersonal communication) influences their attitudes and ongoing behaviors, and how we talk to ourselves (intrapersonal communication) influences our own behavior and attitude. Therefore, this chapter also addresses self-talk — the mental scripts we carry around in our heads before, during, and after our behaviors.

It's fair to say that the nature of our safety-related conversations with others influences degree of involvement in safety. The variety of the safety-related conversations we have with ourselves influences whether we feel accountable to someone else for our safe behaviors or whether we feel self-accountable for our safety-related behaviors. This is the distinction I introduced in Chapter 9 between feeling accountable or other-directed vs. responsible or self-directed.

The bottom line is that I believe the long-term success of any effort to prevent injuries in the workplace, in the home, and on the road is determined by conversation.

The power of conversation

I'm convinced the dramatic success companies experience with behavior-based safety is essentially due to an increase in the quality and quantity of safety correspondence

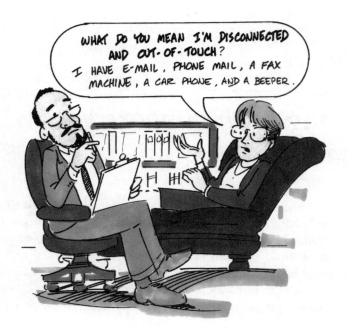

Figure 13.1 The power of conversation comes from face-to-face communication.

— not the high-tech communication referred to in Figure 13.1, but one-on-one interpersonal conversation about safety. Such improvement, in turn, benefits people's self-talk about safety, increasing their sense of personal control and optimism regarding their ability to prevent occupational injuries.

This chapter offers guidelines and techniques for getting more beneficial impact from our conversations with others and with ourselves. Then four types of safety management are presented, each defined by the nature of interpersonal conversation.

The art of improving conversation

Conversation is a powerful tool that shapes personal and team attitudes about loyalty, commitment, social support, and safety. Each of the techniques presented here can get employees more involved in safety, and improve the overall level of workplace safety performance.

Applying these techniques can also improve how you talk to yourself — your "self-talk." The payoff is increased self-esteem and perceptions of empowerment, which are essential for increasing our willingness to actively care for the safety and health of others.

Do not look back

Has this ever happened to you? You ask for more safety involvement from a particular individual and you get a reaction like "I offered a safety suggestion three years ago and no one responded." You may have attended a safety meeting where people spent more time going over past accomplishments or failures than discussing future possibilities and deriving action plans.

These are examples of conversations stuck in the past. The discussion might be enjoyable but little or no progress is made. Conversations about past events help us connect with others and recognize similar experiences, opinions, and motives, but such communication does not enable progress toward problem solving or continuous improvement. For this to happen, the conversation must leave the past and move on.

To direct the flow of a conversation from the past to future possibilities and then to the development of a practical action plan for the present, you first must recognize and appreciate what the other person has to say. Then shift the focus toward the future. Remember, you are approaching this person to discuss possibilities for safety improvement and specific ways to get started now.

Seek commitment

You know your interpersonal conversation is especially productive when someone makes a commitment to improve in a certain way. This reflects success in moving conversation from the past to the future and then to a specific action plan. A verbal commitment also tells you that something is happening on an intrapersonal level within that other person. The person is becoming self-motivated, increasing the probability the target behavior will improve.

Now you can proceed to talk about how that commitment can be supported or how to hold the individual accountable. For example, one person might offer to help a coworker meet an obligation through verbal reminders or an individual might agree to honor a commitment by showing a coach behavioral records that indicate improvement. This is, of course, the kind of follow-up conversation that facilitates personal achievement.

Stop and listen

In their eagerness to prevent injury, safety advocates often give corrective feedback in a top-down, controlling manner. In other words, passion for safety sometimes leads to an overly directive approach to get others to change their behavior. You know from personal experience that a less directive approach to giving advice is often more effective, especially over the long term.

Think about it. How do you respond when someone overtly tells you what to do? Now it certainly depends on who is giving the instruction, but I bet your reaction is not entirely positive. You might follow the instruction, especially if it comes from someone with the power to control consequences, but how will you feel? Will you be motivated to make a permanent change? You might if you asked for the direction, but if you did not request feedback, you could feel insulted or embarrassed.

Corrective feedback interpreted as an "adult-child" confrontation will probably not work. The supervisor in Figure 13.2 means well, but the worker does not see it that way. When a directive conversation is interpreted as controlling or demeaning, it's essentially ineffective, so play it safe. Try to be more nondirective when using interpersonal conversation to affect behavior change.

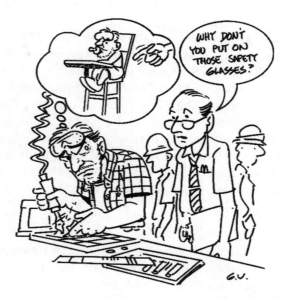

Figure 13.2 Corrective feedback can feel demeaning.

Ask questions first

Instead of telling people what to do, try this. Get them to tell you, in their own words, what they ought to be doing in order to be safe. You can do this by asking questions with a sincere and caring demeanor. Avoid at all costs a sarcastic or demeaning tone and, first, point out certain safe behaviors you noticed — it's important to emphasize positives.

Then move on to the seemingly at-risk behavior by asking, "Is there a safer way to perform that task?" Of course, you hope for more than a "yes" or "no" response to a question like this. However, if that is all you get, you need to be more precise in follow-up questioning. You might, for example, point out a particular work routine that seems risky and ask whether there's a safer way.

I recommend approaching a corrective feedback conversation as if you do not know the safest cooperating procedures, even though you think you do. You might, in fact, find your presumptions to be imperfect. The "expert" on the job might know something you don't know. If you approach the situation with this mindset, you will not get the kind of reaction given by the woman in Figure 13.3.

By asking questions, you are always going to learn something. If nothing else you will hear the rationale behind taking a risk over choosing the safer alternative. You might uncover a barrier to safety that you can help the person overcome. A conversation that entertains ways to remove obstacles that hinder safe behavior is especially valuable if it translates possibilities into feasible and relevant action plans.

You will know your nondirective approach to correction worked if your colleague owns up to his or her mistake even under a cloud of excuses. Remember, it's only natural to offer a rationale for taking a risk. It's a way of protecting self-esteem. Let it pass, and remind yourself that when someone admits a mistake *before* you point it out, there's a greater chance for both acceptance of responsibility and behavior to change.

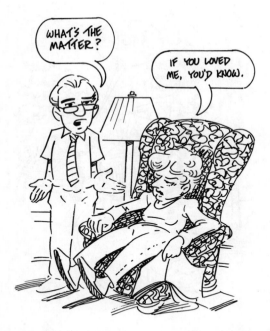

Figure 13.3 Diagnosis requires questions and answers.

Transition from nondirective to directive

What if the person does not give a satisfactory answer to your questions about safer alternatives? What if the individual does not seem to know the safest operating procedure? Now you need to shift the conversation from nondirective to directive. You need to give behavior-focused advice.

In this case, start with a phrase like, "as you know," as my friend John Drebinger (2000) advises. Open the conversation with a phrase that implies the person really does know the safe way to perform, but for some reason just overlooked it (or forgot) this time. This could happen to anyone. Such an opening can help prevent others from feeling their intelligence or safety knowledge has been insulted.

Beware of bias

Every conversation you have with someone is biased by prejudice or prejudgment filters — in yourself and within the other person. You cannot get around it. From personal experience, people develop opinions and attitudes and these, in turn, influence subsequent experience. With regard to interpersonal conversation, we have subjective prejudgment filters that influence what words we hear, how we interpret those words, and what we say in response to those words. In Chapter 5, I referred to this bias as premature cognitive commitment. Every conversation influences how we process and interpret the next conversation.

Figure 13.4 illustrates what I mean. The female driver is merely trying to inform the other driver of an obstacle in the road, but that's not what the driver of the pickup hears. This driver's prior driving experiences lead to a biased interpretation of the warning. You could call such selective listening an "autobiographical bias" (Covey,

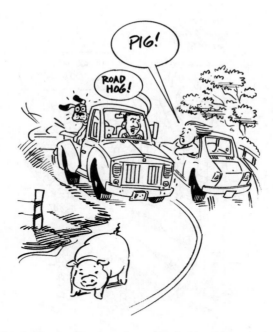

Figure 13.4 Selective listening can be hazardous to your health.

1989). Of course, factors besides prior experience can bias interpersonal communication, including personality, mood state, physiological needs, and future expectations.

It's probably impossible to escape completely the impact of this premature bias in our conversations, but we can exert some control. Actually, each of the conversation strategies discussed here is helpful. For example, the nondirective approach attempts to overcome this bias by listening actively and asking questions before giving instruction. With this approach, a person's biasing filters can be identified and considered in the customization of a plan for corrective action.

Pay close attention to the body language and tone in conversations. I'm sure you have heard many times that the method of delivery can hold as much as or more information than the words themselves. Listen for passion, commitment, or caring. If nothing else, you could learn whether the messenger understands and believes the message and, perhaps, you will learn a new way to deliver a message yourself. The bottom line is our intrapersonal conversations can either facilitate or hinder what we learn from interpersonal conversation.

Recognizing safety achievement

The "Flow of Behavior Change" model presented in Chapter 9 (see Figure 9.6) indicates that supportive intervention through interpersonal recognition is critical for making safe behavior more fluent. Thus, supportive safety conversations are needed throughout a work culture, since most of us need to be more fluent at performing some safety-related behaviors. Yet, this type of conversation is relatively rare.

We're more likely to use our interpersonal conversations to correct rather than support or recognize. In fact, we're more inclined to beat ourselves up for our own

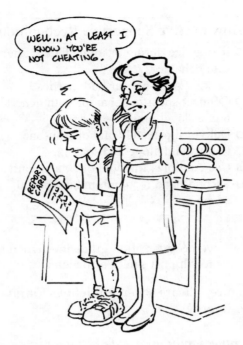

Figure 13.5 Prospect for the good in others.

mistakes, instead of celebrating our personal successes. Now, how can this be explained? Why do we pay more attention to the negative things in our lives?

One reason is the mistakes stick out. They upset the flow and are readily noticed. When people are doing the right thing, the process runs smoothly and we keep on going. We go with the flow. We hardly notice the variety of good behaviors occurring at the time. Instead of being a "good finder," we wait for the obvious mistake and then make our move.

Another reason for our focus on the negative is we've come to believe people learn best by making mistakes. We think paying attention to errors is the best way to improve performance. Behavioral research tells us this is wrong. We learn best when we get positive reinforcement for doing the right thing. As discussed in Chapter 11, positive consequences are good for our attitude. You know how you feel when you get recognition — when it's genuine. You feel good, and that's what we need. We need people feeling good about themselves when they go out of their way for safety.

We need to have the same mindset about safety that the gold prospectors had about their challenge. Their focus was in finding gold. They sifted to find the good, not the bad. Likewise, we need to prospect for the good behaviors, even when the bad might be more obvious. Mom has the right idea in Figure 13.5.

After finding good behavior, it's important to recognize the right way. Most of us have not been taught how to give recognition effectively. Our common sense is not sufficient. Behavioral research, however, has revealed strategies for making interpersonal recognition most rewarding. When you know how to maximize the impact of your recognition, you might use this powerful supportive intervention

> ## How to Give Supportive Recognition
>
> ❏ Recognize during or immediately after safe behavior.
> ❏ Make it personal for both parties.
> ❏ Connect specific behavior with general higher-level praise.
> ❏ Deliver it privately and one-on-one.
> ❏ Let it stand alone and soak in.
> ❏ Use tangibles for symbolic value only.
> ❏ Second-hand recognition has special advantages.

Figure 13.6 Follow seven conversation guidelines when giving recognition to support safety achievement.

more often. Listed in Figure 13.6 are seven guidelines for giving quality recognition. Let's consider each one in order.

Recognize during or immediately after safe behavior

In order for recognition to provide optimal direction and support, it needs to be associated directly with the desired behavior. People need to know what they did to earn the appreciation. If it's necessary to delay the recognition, then the conversation should relive the activity that deserves recognition. Reliving the behavior means talking specifically about what warrants the attention. You could ask the person you are recognizing to describe aspects of the situation and the desirable behavior. This facilitates direction and motivation to continue the behavior. When you connect a person's behavior with recognition you also make the supportive conversation special and personal.

Make recognition personal for both parties

A supportive conversation is most meaningful when it's personal. The recognition should not be general appreciation that could fit anyone in any situation. Rather, it needs to be customized to fit a particular individual and circumstance. This happens, naturally, when the recognition is linked to specific behavior.

When you recognize someone you're expressing personal thanks. It's tempting to say *"we* appreciate" rather than *"I* appreciate" and to refer to company gratitude instead of personal gratitude. Speaking for the company can come across as impersonal and insincere. Of course, it's appropriate to reflect value to the organization when giving praise, but the focus should be personal. "I saw what you did to support our safety process and I really appreciate it. Your example illustrates actively caring and demonstrates the kind of leadership we need around here to achieve a Total Safety Culture." This second statement illustrates the next guideline for giving quality recognition.

Connect specific behavior with general higher-level praise

A supportive conversation is most memorable when it reflects a higher-order characteristic. Adding a universal attitude like leadership, integrity, trustworthiness, or actively caring to the recognition statement makes the recognition more rewarding and most likely to increase the kind of intrapersonal communication that boosts self-esteem. It's important to state the specific behavior first and then make a clear connection between the behavior and the positive attribute it reflects.

Deliver recognition privately and one-on-one

Because quality recognition is personal and indicative of higher-order attributes, it needs to be delivered in private. After all, the recognition is special and only relevant to one person. So, it will mean more and seem more genuine if it's given from one individual to another.

It seems conventional to recognize individuals in front of a group. This approach is typified in athletic contests and reflected in the pop psychology slogan "Praise publicly and reprimand privately." Many managers take the lead from this common-sense statement and give their individual recognition at group meetings. Is it not maximally rewarding to be held up as an exemplar in front of one's peers? Not necessarily — many people feel embarrassed when receiving special attention in a group.

Let recognition stand alone and soak in

Keep a supportive conversation simple and to the point. Give your behavior-based praise a chance to soak in. In this fast-paced age of trying to do more with less, we try to communicate as much as possible when we finally get in touch with a busy person. After recognizing a person's special safety effort, we are tempted to tag on a bunch of unrelated statements, even a request for additional behavior. This comes across as, "I appreciate what you've done for safety, but I need more." Resist the temptation to do more than praise the good behavior you saw. If you have additional points to discuss, it's better to reconnect later, after your praise has had a chance to sink in and become a part of the person's self-talk.

Use tangibles for symbolic value only

Tangibles can detract from the self-motivation aspect of quality recognition. If the focus of a recognition process is placed on a material reward, the words of appreciation can seem less significant. In turn, the impact on one's intrapersonal conversation system is lessened.

On the other hand, tangibles can add to the quality of interpersonal recognition if they are delivered as tokens of appreciation. As discussed in Chapter 11, if tangibles include a safety slogan, they can help to promote safety. But how you deliver a trinket will determine whether it adds to or subtracts from the value of your supportive conversation. The benefit of your praise is weakened if the tangible is viewed as a payoff for the safety-related behavior. On the other hand, if the tangible is seen as symbolic of going beyond the call of duty for safety, it strengthens the praise.

Secondhand recognition has special advantages

Up to this point, I have been discussing one-on-one verbal conversation in which one person recognizes another person directly for a particular safety-related behavior. It's also possible to recognize a person's outstanding efforts indirectly; such an approach can have special benefits. Suppose, for example, you overhear me talk to another person about your outstanding safety presentation. How will this secondhand recognition affect you? Will you believe my words of praise were genuine?

Sometimes people are suspicious of the genuineness of praise when it's delivered face-to-face. The receiver of praise might feel, for example, there's an ulterior motive to the recognition. The deliverer of praise might be expecting a favor in return for the special recognition. Perhaps both individuals have recently attended the same behavior-based safety course, and the verbal exchange is viewed as only an extension of a communication exercise. It, thus, will be devalued as sincere appreciation. Secondhand recognition, however, is not as easily tainted with these potential biases. Therefore, its genuineness is less suspect.

My point here is that gossip can be good — *if it is positive*. When we talk about the success of others in behavior-specific terms, we begin a cycle of positive communication that can support desired behavior. It also helps to build an internal script for self-motivation. We also set an example for the kind of inter- and intrapersonal conversations that increase self-esteem, empowerment, and group cohesion. As explained in Part 5 of this book, these are the very person states that increase actively caring behaviors and cultivate the achievement of a Total Safety Culture.

Receiving recognition well

The list of guidelines for giving quality recognition is not exhaustive, but it does cover the basics. Following these guidelines will increase the benefit of a conversation to support desirable performance. The most important point is that more recognition for safe behavior is needed in every organization, whether given firsthand or indirectly through positive gossip. It only takes a few seconds to deliver quality recognition.

Most of us get so little recognition from others we are caught completely off guard when acknowledged for our actions. We do not know how to accept appreciation when it finally comes. Some claim they do not deserve the special recognition. Others actually accuse the person giving recognition of being insincere or wanting something from them. This can be quite embarrassing to the person doing the recognizing. It could certainly discourage that person from giving more recognition.

Remember the basic motivational principle that consequences influence the behaviors they follow. Well, this is true for both the person giving recognition and the person receiving recognition. Quality recognition increases the behavior being recognized and one's reaction to the recognition influences whether the recognizing behavior is likely to occur again. Thus, it's crucial to react appropriately when we receive recognition from others. Seven basic guidelines for receiving recognition are listed in Figure 13.7. Here's an explanation for each.

How to Receive Supportive Recognition

❏ Avoid denial and disclaimer statements.
❏ Listen actively with genuine appreciation.
❏ Relive recognition later for self-motivation.
❏ Show sincere appreciation.
❏ Recognize the person for recognizing you.
❏ Embrace the reciprocity principle.
❏ Ask for recognition when it is deserved but
   not forthcoming.

Figure 13.7 Follow seven converation guidelines when receiving recognition
in order to increase the occurrence of interpersonal support.

Avoid denial and disclaimer statements

Whenever I attempt to give quality recognition, whether to a colleague, student, waitress, hotel clerk, or a member of the baseball team I coach, the most common reaction I get is awkward denial. Some act as if they did not hear me and keep doing whatever they are doing, or they offer a disclaimer like "It really was nothing special," "Just doing my job," "I really could not have done it without your support," or "Other members of our team deserve more credit than I."

We need to accept recognition without denial and disclaimer statements and we should not deflect the credit to others. It's okay to show pride in our small-win accomplishments, even if others contributed to the successful outcome. After all, the vision of a Total Safety Culture includes everyone going beyond the call of duty for their own safety and that of others. In this context, most people deserve recognition on a daily basis. It's not "employee of the month," it's "employee of the moment."

Listen attentively with genuine appreciation

Listen proactively to the person giving you recognition. You want to know what you did right. Plus, you can evaluate whether the recognition is given well. If the recognition does not pinpoint a particular behavior, you might ask the person, "What did I do to deserve this?" This will help to improve that person's method of giving recognition.

Of course, it's important not to seem critical but rather to show genuine appreciation for the special attention. Consider how difficult it is for most people to go out of their way to recognize others. Then revel in the fact you are receiving some recognition, even if its quality could be improved. Remember that a person who recognizes you is showing gratitude for what you do and will come to like you more if you accept the recognition well.

Relive recognition later for self-motivation

Obviously, most of your safety-related behaviors go unnoticed. You perform many of these when no one else is around to observe you. Even when other people are available, they will likely be so preoccupied with their own routines they will not notice your extra effort. So when you finally do receive some recognition, take it in as well-deserved. Remember the many times you have gone the extra mile for safety but did not get noticed.

You need to listen intently to every word of praise, not only to show you care but also because you want to remember this special occasion. Relive this moment later by talking to yourself. Such self-recognition can motivate you to continue going beyond the call of duty for safety.

Show sincere appreciation

After listening actively with humble acceptance, you need to show sincere gratitude with a smile and a "thank you." As I have already emphasized, your reaction to being recognized can determine whether similar recognition will occur again. So be prepared to say something to reflect pleasure in the special conversation. I find it natural to add "You've made my day," to a "Thank you" because it's the truth. When people go out of their way to offer me quality recognition, they *have* made my day and I often relive such situations to improve a later day.

Recognize the person for recognizing you

When you accept recognition well, you reward the person giving support for their extra effort. This can motivate that individual to do more recognizing. Sometimes, you can do even more to increase quality recognition. Specifically, you can recognize the person for recognizing you. In this case, you apply quality recognition principles to reward certain aspects of the supportive conversation. You might say, for example, you really appreciate the pinpointing of a certain behavior and the reference to higher-order praise. Such rewarding feedback provides direction and motivation for those aspects of the recognition process that are especially worthwhile and need to become habitual.

Embrace the reciprocity principle

Some people resist receiving recognition because they do not want to feel obligated to give recognition to others. This is the reciprocity norm at work. If we want to cultivate a Total Safety Culture, we need to embrace this norm. Research has shown that when you are nice to others, as when providing them with special praise, you increase the likelihood they will reciprocate by showing similar behavior. You might not receive the returned favor, but someone will.

The bottom line is to realize your genuine acceptance of quality recognition will activate the reciprocity norm, and the more this norm is activated from positive interpersonal conversation, the greater the frequency of interpersonal recognition. So accept recognition well and embrace the reciprocity norm. The result will be more interpersonal involvement consistent with the vision of a Total Safety Culture.

Ask for recognition when deserved but not forthcoming

There is one final strategy I'd like to recommend for increasing recognition conversation throughout a culture. If you feel you deserve recognition, why not ask for it? This might result in recognition viewed as less genuine than if it were spontaneous, but the outcome from such a request can be quite beneficial. You might receive some words worth reliving later for self-motivation. Most important, you will remind the other individual in a nice way that he or she missed a prime opportunity to offer quality recognition. This could be a valuable learning experience for that person.

Consider the possible benefit from your statement to another person that you are pleased with a certain result of your extra effort. With the right tone and effect, such verbal behavior will not seem like bragging but rather a declaration of personal pride in a small-win accomplishment. The other person will probably support your personal praise with individual testimony, and this will bolster your own self-motivation. Plus, you'll teach the other person how to support the safety-related behaviors of others.

In conclusion

I hope I've convinced you that the status of safety in your organization is greatly determined by how safety is talked about — from the managers' board room to the workers' break room. Whether we feel responsible for safety and are committed to go for a breakthrough depends on our interpretations or mental scripts about safety conversation.

We often focus our interpersonal and intrapersonal conversations on the past. This helps us connect with others, but it also feeds our prejudice filters and limits the potential for conversation to facilitate beneficial change. We enable progress when we move conversations with ourselves and others from past to future possibilities and then to the development of an action plan.

Expect people to protect their self-esteem with excuses for their past mistakes. Listen proactively for barriers to safe behavior reflected in these excuses. Then help the conversation shift to a discussion of possibilities for improvement and personal commitment to apply a feasible action plan. This is often more likely to occur with a nondirective than directive approach in which more questions are asked than directives given. It's also useful to use opening words to protect the listener's self-esteem and limit the impact of reactive bias.

Remember that everyone needs genuine recognition now and then for doing the right thing, especially when they do it for safety. Following the guidelines given here for delivering and receiving quality recognition will increase the frequency of such supportive conversation and its interpersonal and intrapersonal benefits. William James, the first renowned American psychologist, wrote "the deepest principle in human nature is the craving to be appreciated" (from Carnegie, 1936, page 19).

part five

Actively caring for safety

chapter fourteen

Understanding actively caring

Actively caring is planned and purposeful behavior, directed at environment, person, or behavior factors. It's reactive or proactive and direct or indirect. Direct, proactive, and behavior-focused actively caring is most challenging, but it is usually most important for large-scale injury prevention. This chapter discusses conditions and situations that inhibit actively caring behavior. We need to understand why people resist opportunities to actively care for safety. Then, we can develop interventions to increase this desired behavior which is critical for achieving a Total Safety Culture.

"We cannot live only for ourselves. A thousand fibers connect us with our fellow men; and among those fibers, as sympathetic threads, our actions run as causes; and they come back to us as effects." — Herman Melville

This quotation from Herman Melville appeared in a popular paperback entitled *Random Acts of Kindness* (page 31). Here, the editors of Conari Press (1993) introduced the idea of randomly showing kindness or generosity toward others for no ulterior motive except to benefit humanity. This notion seems quite analogous to the actively caring concept I have discussed earlier in various contexts. Indeed, a recurring theme in this book is that a Total Safety Culture can only be achieved if people intervene regularly to protect and promote the safety and health of others. Actively caring, however, is not usually random. It is planned and purposeful; plus, as implied in Melville's quote, actively caring behaviors (actions) are supported by positive consequences (effects).

Part 5 of this book addresses the need to increase actively caring behavior throughout a culture and to get the maximum safety and health benefits from this type of behavioral intervention. Psychologists have identified conditions and individual characteristics (or person states) that influence people's willingness to actively care for the safety or health of others. I'll present these and link them to practical things we can do to increase the occurrence of active caring.

What is actively caring?

Figure 14.1 presents a simple flow chart summarizing the basic approach to culture change. We start a culture-change mission with a vision or ultimate purpose — for

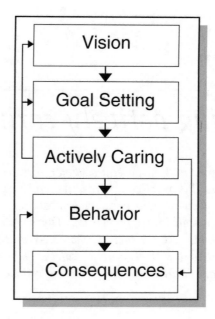

Figure 14.1 Continuous improvement requires actively caring.

example, to achieve a Total Safety Culture. With group consensus supporting the vision, we develop procedures or action plans to accomplish our mission. These are reflected in process-oriented goals, which, we hope, activate goal-related behaviors.

Appropriate goal setting (as I described in Chapter 10), self-affirmations, and a positive attitude can activate behaviors to achieve goals and visions, but we must not forget one of Skinner's most important legacies — "selection by consequences" (Skinner, 1981). As depicted in Figure 14.1, consequences are needed to support the right behaviors and correct wrong ones. Without support for the "right stuff," good intentions and initial efforts fade away. Sometimes, natural consequences are available to motivate desired behaviors, but often — especially in safety — consequences need to be managed to motivate the behavior needed to achieve our goals.

However, vision, goals, and consequences are not sufficient for culture change. People need to actively care about goals, action plans, and consequences. They need to believe in and own the vision. They need to feel obligated to work toward attaining goals that support the vision, and they need to give rewarding or corrective feedback to increase behaviors consistent with vision-relevant goals. This is the key to continuous improvement and to achieving a Total Safety Culture.

Three ways to actively care

The "Safety Triad" introduced in Chapter 3 is useful to categorize actively caring behaviors. These behaviors can address environment factors, person factors, or behaviors. When people alter environmental conditions or reorganize or redistribute resources in an attempt to benefit others, they are actively caring from an environment perspective. Behaviors in this category include attending to housekeeping details, posting a warning sign near an environmental hazard, designing a guard for a machine, locking out the energy source to production equipment, and cleaning up a spill.

Person-based actively caring occurs when we attempt to make other people feel better. We address their emotions, attitudes, or mood states. Proactively listening to others, inquiring with concern about another person's difficulties, complimenting an individual's personal appearance, and sending a get-well card are examples. This type of active caring is likely to boost a person's self-esteem, optimism, or sense of belonging — which, in turn, increases one's propensity to actively care. I discuss this in detail in Chapter 15, as well as reactive behaviors performed in crisis situations. For example, if you pull someone out of an equipment pinch point or administer cardiopulmonary resuscitation, you're actively caring from a person-based perspective.

From a proactive perspective, behavior-based actively caring is most constructive and most challenging. This happens when you apply an instructive, supportive, or motivational intervention to improve another person's safe behavior. Obviously, the one-on-one coaching process described in Chapter 12 represents behavior-based actively caring. Giving someone behavior-based recognition in a supportive conversation, as discussed in Chapter 13, is also actively caring with a behavior focus.

Why categorize actively caring behaviors?

So why go to the trouble of categorizing actively caring behaviors? Good question! I think it's useful to consider what these behaviors are trying to accomplish and to realize the relative difficulty in performing each of them. Environment-focused caring might be easiest for some people because it usually does not involve interpersonal interaction. When people contribute to a charity, donate blood, or complete an organ donor card, they don't interact personally with the recipient of the contribution. These behaviors are certainly commendable and may represent significant commitment and effort, but the absence of personal encounters between giver and receiver warrants consideration separate from other types of actively caring behavior.

Certain conditions and personality traits might facilitate or inhibit one type of actively caring behavior and not the other. For example, communication skills are needed to actively care on the personal or behavioral level and different skills usually come into play. Behavior-focused active caring is more direct and usually more intrusive than person-focused caring. It's riskier and potentially more confrontational to attempt to direct or motivate another person's behavior than it is to demonstrate concern, respect, or empathy for someone.

Classifying actively caring behaviors also provides insight into their benefits and liabilities. Both Brown (1991) and the editors of Conari Press (1993) recommend we feed expired parking meters to keep people from paying excessive fines. Let's consider the behavioral impact of this environment-focused "random act of kindness." What will the vehicle owner think when finding an unexpired parking meter? Could this lead to a belief that parking meters are unreliable — and further mismanagement of time? Is there a price to pay for people becoming less responsible about sharing public parking spaces?

When considering the long-term and large-scale impact of some actively caring strategies, other approaches might come to mind. In the parking meter situation, for example, the potential impact would be improved by adding some behavior-focused actively caring. Along with feeding the expired parking meter, why not place a note under the vehicle's windshield wiper explaining the act? The note might also include some time management hints. This additional step might not only improve behavior, but set an example. The recipient of the note is probably more inclined to actively care for someone else.

Each type of actively caring behavior can be direct or indirect, with direct behavior requiring effective communication strategies. For instance, leaving a note to explain an actively caring act does not involve interpersonal conversation. Similarly, you can report an individual's safe or at-risk behavior to a supervisor and eliminate the need for one-on-one communication skills.

In the same vein, person-focused actively caring does not always involve inter-personal dialogue. You can send someone a get-well card or leave a friendly uplifting statement on an answering machine or by e-mail. It is also possible that environment-focused acts will include personal confrontation, say, if you deliver a contribution to a needy individual. This additional category for actively caring behavior is illustrated in Figure 14.2.

An illustrative anecdote

Several years ago, I was driving on a toll road in Norfolk, VA, en route to the Fort Eustis Army Base, where a transportation safety conference was being held. Of my students, three were with me. Each was scheduled to give a 15-minute talk at the conference. This was to be their first professional presentation and they appeared quite distressed. Each was paging frantically through his or her notes making last-minute adjustments.

> "Were you this nervous, Doc, when you gave your first professional address?" one student asked.
> "No, I don't think so," I replied in jest. " I was obviously better prepared."
> "Can we just read our paper?" asked another.
> "Absolutely not," I retorted. "Anyone could read your paper. It's much more professional and instructive to just talk about your paper informally with the audience."

Naturally, this conversation just caused more anxiety and distress for my students. Something had to be done to distract them — to break the tension. As we approached the first of several toll booths along the highway, I thought of an actively caring solution. After paying a quarter for my vehicle, I handed the attendant another quarter and said, "This is for the vehicle behind us; the driver is using a safety belt and deserves the recognition." My students put down their papers and watched the attendant explain to the driver that we paid her toll because she was buckled up. Because we slowed down to observe this, the driver caught up with us, pulled next to us in the right lane, and acknowledged our actively caring behavior with a "shoul-der belt salute" — a smile and tug on her shoulder strap.

At the next toll booth, the driver of the vehicle behind us was not buckled up, but that did not stop me. I gave the attendant an extra quarter and said, "This is for the vehicle behind us; please ask the driver to buckle up." Again, we slowed down

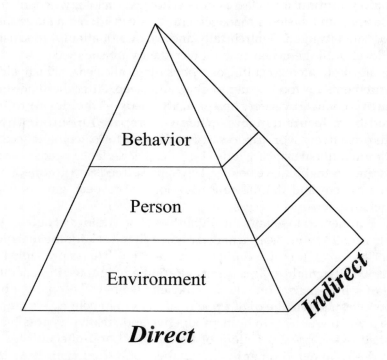

Figure 14.2 Actively caring is usually most challenging and useful
when direct and behavior-focused.

to watch and, to our delight, the driver buckled up on the spot. When the vehicle passed us, the driver gave us a smile and a "thumbs up" sign.

I kept doing this at every toll booth until exiting the highway, by which time my students had almost forgotten about their papers. They seemed relaxed and at ease when entering the conference room and each gave an excellent presentation. Later, we discussed how the toll booth intervention took their minds off their papers and their anxiety.

Brown (1991) recommended that his son occasionally pay the toll for the vehicle behind him. This is redistribution of resources. It is also actively caring with an environment focus. By adding a safety-belt message, I was able to accomplish more than the "random act of kindness" suggested by Brown (1991) and the Editors of Conari Press (1993). I was able to support those who were already buckled up and to influence some drivers to buckle up. In other words, realizing the special value of behavior-based actively caring enabled me to get more benefit from an environment-focused strategy with very little extra effort. This behavior-based effort was particularly convenient and effortless because it was indirect. You can see how the system for categorizing actively caring behavior allows us to compare real and potential acts of kindness and then to consider ways to increase their impact.

A hierarchy of needs

The hierarchy of needs proposed by the humanist Abraham Maslow (1943) is probably the most popular theory of human motivation. It is taught in a variety of college courses, including introductory classes in psychology, sociology, economics, marketing, human factors, and systems management. It is considered a stage theory. Categories of needs are arranged hierarchically and we do not attempt to satisfy needs at one stage or level until the needs at the lower stages are satisfied.

First, we are motivated to fulfill our physiological needs, which include basic survival requirements for food, water, shelter, and sleep. After these needs are under control, we are motivated by safety and security needs — the desire to feel secure and protected from future dangers. When we prepare for future physiological needs, we are proactively working to satisfy our need for safety and security.

The next motivational stage includes our social acceptance needs — the need to have friends and to feel like we belong. When these needs are gratified, our concern focuses on self-esteem and the desire to develop self-respect, gain the approval of others, and achieve personal success.

When I ask audiences to tell me the highest level of Maslow's Hierarchy of Needs, several people usually shout "self-actualization." When I ask for the meaning of "self-actualization," however, I receive limited or no reaction. This is probably because the concept of being self-actualized is rather vague and ambiguous. In general terms, we reach a level of self-actualization when we believe we have become the best we can be, taking the fullest advantage of our potential as human beings. We are working to reach this level when we strive to be as productive and creative as possible. Once this is accomplished, we possess a feeling of brotherhood and affection for all human beings and a desire to help humanity as members of a single family — the human race. Perhaps it's fair to say that these individuals are ready to actively care.

Maslow's Hierarchy of Needs is illustrated in Figure 14.3, but self-actualization is not at the top. Maslow (1971) revised his renowned hierarchy shortly before his death to put self-transcendence above self-actualization. Transcending the self means going beyond self-interest and is quite analogous to the actively caring concept. According to Viktor Frankl (1962), for example, self-transcendence includes giving ourselves to a cause or another person and is the ultimate state of existence for the healthy person. Thus, after satisfying needs for self-preservation, safety and security, acceptance, self-esteem, and self-actualization, people can be motivated to reach the ultimate state of self-transcendence by reaching out to help others — to actively care.

The psychology of actively caring

Walking home on March 13, 1964, Catherine (Kitty) Genovese reached her apartment in Queens, NY, at 3:30 a.m. Suddenly, a man approached with a knife, stabbed her repeatedly, and then raped her. When Kitty screamed, "Oh my God, he stabbed me! Please help me!" into the early morning stillness, lights went on and windows opened in nearby buildings. Seeing the lights, the attacker fled, but when he saw no one come to the victim's aid, he returned to stab her eight more times and rape her again. The murder and rape lasted more than 30 minutes and was witnessed by 38 neighbors. One couple pulled up chairs to their window and turned off their lights so they could get a better view. Only after the murderer and rapist departed for good did anyone phone the police. When the neighbors were questioned about their lack of intervention, they could not explain it.

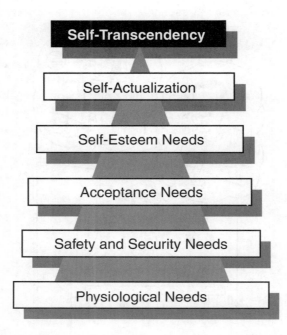

Figure 14.3 The highest need in Maslow's hierarchy reflects actively caring.

Lessons from research

Professors Bibb Latané and John Darley and their colleagues (1970) studied bystander apathy by staging emergency events observed by varying numbers of individuals. Then, they systematically recorded the speed at which one or more persons came to the victim's rescue. In the most controlled experiments, the observers sat in separate cubicles (as depicted in Figure 14.4) and could not be influenced by the body language of other subjects. In the first study of this type, the subjects introduced themselves and discussed problems associated with living in an urban environment. In each condition, the first individual introduced himself and then casually mentioned he had epilepsy and that the pressures of city life made him prone to seizures. During the course of the discussion over the intercom, he became increasingly loud and incoherent, choking, gasping, and crying out before lapsing into silence. The experimenters measured how quickly the subjects left their cubicles to help him.

When subjects believed they were the only witness, 85 percent left their cubicles within three minutes to intervene. However, only 62 percent of the subjects who believed one other witness was present left their cubicle to intervene, and only 31 percent of those who thought five other witnesses were available attempted to intervene. Within three to six minutes after the seizure began, 100 percent of the lone subjects, 81 percent of the subjects with one presumed witness, and 62 percent of the subjects with five other bystanders left their cubicles to intervene.

The reduced tendency of observers of an emergency to help a victim when they believe other potential helpers are available has been termed the *bystander effect* and has been replicated in several situations. Researchers have systematically explored

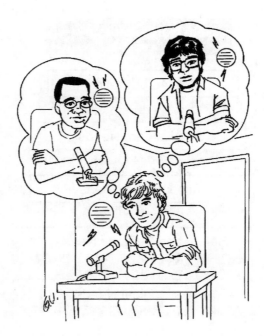

Figure 14.4 Subjects in the Latané and Darley experiment could not see each other and thought they were conversing with one, two, or five other individuals.

reasons for the bystander effect and have identified conditions influencing this phenomenon. The results most relevant to safety management are reviewed here.

Diffusion of responsibility. It is likely many observers of the Kitty Genovese rape and murder assumed that another witness would call the police or attempt to scare away the assailant. Perhaps, some observers waited for a witness more capable than they to rescue Kitty. Does this factor contribute to lack of intervention for occupational safety? Do people overlook environmental hazards or at-risk behaviors in the workplace because they presume someone else will make the correction? Perhaps some people assume, "If the employees who work in the work area don't care enough to remove the hazard or correct the risk, why should I?"

A helping norm. Many, if not most, U.S. citizens are raised to be independent rather than interdependent. However, intervening for the benefit of others, whether reactively in a crisis situation or proactively to prevent a crisis, requires sincere belief and commitment toward interdependence. Social psychologists refer to a "social responsibility norm" as the belief that people should help those who need help. Subjects who scored high on a measure of this norm, as a result of upbringing during childhood or special training sessions, were more likely to intervene in a bystander intervention study, regardless of the number of other witnesses.

Knowing what to do. When people know what to do in a crisis, they do not fear making fools of themselves and do not wait for another, more appropriate person to intervene. The bystander effect was eliminated when observers had certain competencies, such as training in first-aid treatment, which enabled them to take charge of the situation. In other words, when observers believed they had the appropriate tools to help, bystander apathy was decreased or eliminated.

This conclusion is also relevant for proactive or preventive action, as in safety intervention. When people receive tools to improve safety, and believe the tools will be accepted and effective to prevent injuries, bystander apathy for safety will decrease. This implies, of course, the need to promote a social responsibility or interdependence norm throughout the culture, and to teach and support specific intervention strategies or tools to prevent workplace injuries.

It's important to belong. Researchers demonstrated reduced bystander apathy when observers knew one another and had developed a sense of belonging or mutual respect from prior interactions. Most, if not all, of the witnesses to Kitty Genovese's murder did not know her personally and it's likely the neighbors did not feel a sense of comradeship or community with one another. Situations and interactions that reduce a we–they, or territorial, perspective and increase feelings of togetherness or "community" will increase the likelihood of people looking out for each other.

Mood states. Several social psychology studies have found that people are more likely to offer help when they are in a good mood. The mood states that facilitated helping behavior were created very easily — by arranging for potential helpers to find a dime in a phone booth, giving them a cookie, showing them a comedy film, or providing pleasant aromas. Are these findings relevant for occupational safety?

Daily events can elevate or depress our moods. Some events are controllable, some are not. Clearly, the nature of our interactions with others can have a dramatic impact on the mood of everyone involved. Perhaps, remembering the research on mood and its effect will motivate us to adjust our interpersonal conversations with coworkers (see Chapter 13). We should also interact in a way that could influence a person's beliefs or expectations in certain directions, as explained next.

A consequence analysis of actively caring

When I related the Kitty Genovese incident to my family and asked their opinions, I received a unanimous reaction that reflects the influence of consequences — a common theme throughout this book. My wife and two daughters proclaimed that most observers did not help this woman because they feared for their own safety. The perpetrator was armed with a knife. The onlookers could certainly see there was an emergency requiring specific assistance from anyone who would take responsibility.

According to an interpretation based on our understanding of the power of consequences, people resisted taking responsibility because they perceived that it could mean more trouble — or potential harm — than it was worth. It was safer to assume that someone else more capable would intervene. According to this consequence model, people hesitated to intervene because they perceived more potential costs than benefits, not because they were apathetic.

The matrix in Figure 14.5 combines two levels of cost (low vs. high) to the potential intervention agent and the victim in order to predict when actively caring behavior will occur. It's most likely (lower left cell of Figure 14.5) when costs for helping are low, for example, convenient, and not dangerous, and costs to the victim for not helping are high, as when the victim is seriously injured. On the other hand, intervention is least likely when the perceived personal costs for intervening are high, for example, effortful, and risky, and the apparent costs to the victim for no intervention

		Costs to Bystander for Intervening	
		Low	*High*
Costs to Victim for Not Intervening	*Low*	Depends on person factors	Intervention improbable
	High	Intervention probable	Diffusion of responsibility

Figure 14.5 Costs to bystanders for intervening and cost to a victim for not intervening determine the probability of intervention. Adapted from Piliavin et al. (1981).

are low, as when an experienced worker is performing at-risk behavior with no negative consequences.

The Genovese incident fits the lower right cell of Figure 14.5 — high perceived cost for both helper and victim. Although the costs for not helping Kitty were extremely high, resulting ultimately in her death, the costs for helping were also high, in fact, potentially fatal. This means significant conflict for the person deciding what to do. The conflict can be resolved by helping indirectly, say by telephoning police or an ambulance, or by reinterpreting the situation. This can be done by presuming someone else will intervene — diffusion of responsibility — or perhaps by rationalizing that the person does not deserve help.

A bystander might rationalize, for example, that Genovese should not have been walking the streets in that neighborhood at 3:30 in the morning. Rationalization reduces the perceived costs for not intervening and enables the bystander to ignore the situation without excessive shame or guilt. According to this cost-reward interpretation, when bystanders perceive high costs both for intervening and for not intervening in a crisis, they recognize the need for action, hesitate because of perceived personal costs, and then search for an excuse to do nothing, as depicted in Figure 14.6.

The upper left quadrant of Figure 14.5 represents situations most analogous to actively caring for injury prevention. Although a simple low-cost intervention might be called for to correct an environmental hazard or an at-risk behavior, there is no immediate emergency and, thus, no need for immediate action. There's low perceived cost if no action is taken: "We've been working under these conditions for months and no one has been hurt." Intervention in situations represented by this cost quadrant is most difficult to predict. Many factors can influence perceived consequences that are positive and negative, and small changes in these factors can tilt the cost-reward balance in favor of stepping in or standing back.

Through testimonials and constructive discussions, employees can be convinced that the potential cost of not intervening is higher than they initially thought. This can occur, for example, by considering the large degree of plant-wide exposure to a certain uncorrected hazard. Also, it might be worthwhile to remind people of the

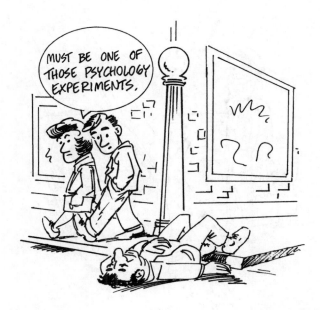

Figure 14.6 People give a variety of excuses for not helping.

large-scale detrimental learning that could occur from the continuous performance of risky behavior. Furthermore, education and role-playing exercises can reduce the perceived person costs of actively caring. It's also true that personal factors, such as mood states discussed earlier, determine whether intervention occurs.

The power of context

The influence of context in determining whether we actually care for another person's safety cannot be overemphasized. The context in which behavior occurs can affect one's evaluation of the costs and benefits of helping vs. not helping a victim. In other words, the perceived consequences of actively caring depend to a significant extent on the environmental and social context in which the relevant behaviors occur. Let's look more closely at this context variable, and consider its impact on safety-related behavior.

According to my copy of *The American Heritage Dictionary* (1991), context refers to "the circumstances in which a particular event occurs" (page 316). It includes both the outside and inside stuff surrounding people when they are performing. This refers to what we see others doing on the outside and how we feel on the inside — from feelings of competence, confidence, and commitment to perceptions of insecurity, uncertainty, and risk.

Figure 14.7 is worth more than a thousand words to describe context. Have you seen a mild-mannered and polite person turn into an impatient and hostile creature after getting behind the wheel of an automobile? The environmental and competitive context of driving interacts with certain personality characteristics to produce "Mr. Hyde" on the road. Then, we have a nationwide epidemic of "road rage."

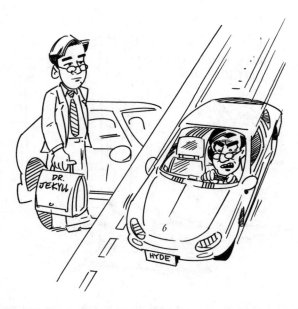

Figure 14.7 In the context of driving, many individuals transition
from mild-mannered to rude, hostile, and impolite.

Context at work

Does the mission statement of your industry reflect an overarching concern for production and quality? Is safety considered a priority (instead of a value) that gets
shifted when production quotas are emphasized? Is safety viewed as a top-down
condition of employment rather than an employee-driven process supported by management? Are safety programs handed down to employees with directives to "implement per instructions" rather than "customize for your own work area"?

Are safety initiatives discussed as short-term "flavor-of-the-month" programs
rather than an ongoing process that needs to be continuously improved to remain
evergreen? Are near-hit and injury "investigations" perceived as fault-finding searches
for a single cause rather than fact-finding opportunities to learn what else can be done
to reduce the probability of personal injury? Are the elements of a safety initiative
considered piecemeal factors independent of other organizational functions rather
than aspects of an organizational system of interdependent functions?

Are employees held accountable for outcome numbers that hold little direction
for proactive change and personal control rather than process numbers that are diagnostic regarding achieving an injury-free workplace? Do employees take a depen-
dency stance toward industrial safety whereby they depend on the organization to
protect them with rules, regulations, engineering safeguards, and personal protective
equipment?

A "yes" answer to any of these questions implies contextual barriers that need to
be overcome in order to achieve the ultimate injury-free workplace. A "no" answer
to all of these questions is symptomatic of a work context that encourages people to
actively care for the health and safety of others. In this kind of work culture, it's not

sufficient to rely on the organization's safe operating procedures or even on personal responsibility and self-discipline, but on interpersonal teamwork and a shared interdependent responsibility to protect each other. In this work context, actively caring can be cultivated and a Total Safety Culture achieved.

In conclusion

Actively caring behavior is planned and purposeful. It can be direct or indirect and its focus is environment, person, or behavior. Actively caring that addresses the environment is usually easiest to perform because it does not require interpersonal confrontation. Behavior-focused actively caring is often most proactive but is most difficult to carry out effectively because it attempts to influence another person's behavior in a nonemergency situation.

The finding that people often refuse to help in a crisis, especially when they can share the responsibility of intervening with others, is quite analogous to most work settings. Hence, it's important to understand the factors that can influence this resistance, referred to as "bystander apathy." For example, people with a sense of social responsibility and comradeship for others at work, and who believe they have personal control in a just world, are more apt to intervene for the safety of others. It's possible to increase these person characteristics among people through policy, procedures, and interpersonal communication. Increasing these states, and thus the willingness to actively care for safety, is key to achieving a Total Safety Culture and is addressed in the next two chapters.

chapter fifteen

The person-based approach to actively caring

Our willingness to actively care for others is affected by certain feelings and states of mind. If we have a strong sense of self-esteem, self-efficacy, personal control, optimism, and belonging, there is a greater chance we will go beyond the call of duty. Each of these person states is explained in this chapter and the research supporting direct relationships between these states and actively caring behavior is reviewed. Understanding these connections enables us to design conditions and interventions to increase actively caring behavior throughout an organization or community.

"Our deeds determine us, as much as we determine our deeds." — George Eliot

This quotation by George Eliot indicates that our behaviors influence something about us and implies that good deeds or actively caring behaviors are good for us. They change something about us and this, in turn, affects subsequent behavior. Does this mean our actively caring behaviors influence us to actively care even more? It's a nice thought and seems intuitive, but what does it really mean?

This chapter explores a host of questions arising from the concept reflected in Eliot's words. What is it about us that changes as a result of our good deeds, and will this change lead to more good deeds? Can making people more willing to actively care be influenced in ways other than managing activators and consequences to directly change behavior? In other words, can we change something inside people that will make them more willing to actively care for the safety and health of others? If answers to these questions can be turned into practical procedures, we will know how to increase actively caring behaviors throughout a culture.

Actively caring from the inside

Perhaps you recall earlier discussions in this text about "outside" vs. "inside" aspects of people. In Chapter 3, for example, I distinguished behaviors (outside) vs. intentions, attitudes, and values (inside), and emphasized that we should start with behaviors. A prime principle of behavior-based psychology is that it's easier, especially for large-scale culture change, to "act a person into safe thinking" than it is to address attitudes and values directly in an attempt to "think a person into safe acting." Another key principle of behavior-based psychology is that the consequences of our behavior influence how we feel about the behavior. Generally, positive consequences lead to good feelings or attitudes; negative consequences lead to bad feelings or attitudes.

Long-term behavior change requires people to change inside as well as outside. The promise of a positive consequence or the threat of a negative one can maintain the desired behavior while the response–consequence contingencies are in place. What happens when they are withdrawn? What happens when people are in situations, like at home, when no one is holding them accountable for their behavior? If people do not *believe* in the safe way of doing something and do not *accept* safety as a value or a personal mission, do not count on them to choose the safe way when they have the choice. In addition, if people are not self-motivated to keep themselves safe, do not expect them to actively care for the safety of others.

As discussed in Chapter 5, numerous internal and situational factors influence how we perceive activators and consequences. For example, if we see activators and consequences as nongenuine ploys to control us, our attitude about the situation will be negative. If we believe the external contingencies are genuine attempts to help us do the right thing, our attitude will be more positive. Thus, personal or internal dynamics determine how we receive activator and consequence information. This can influence whether environmental events enhance or diminish what we do.

In Chapters 10 and 11, I showed how direct manipulations of activators and consequences can influence behavior on a large scale. Now, let's see if changes in internal person factors can benefit behavior change. In particular, how do inside or person factors affect actively caring for safety?

Person traits vs. states

Some person factors are presumed to be *traits*, while others are *states*. Theoretically, traits are relatively permanent characteristics of people and do not vary appreciably over time or across situations. In contrast, states are characteristics that can change moment-to-moment depending on circumstances and personal interactions. When our goals are thwarted, for example, we can be in a state of frustration. When experience leads us to believe we have little control over events around us, we can be in a state of apathy or helplessness. These states can influence certain behaviors.

Frustration often provokes aggressive behavior; perceptions of helplessness can inhibit constructive behavior or facilitate inactivity. In contrast, certain life experiences can affect positive person states, such as optimism, personal control, self-confidence, and a sense of belonging. This, in turn, increases constructive behavior, including actively caring.

Actively caring states

I contend that actively caring characteristics internal to people are states, not traits. Plus, certain conditions — including activators and consequences — can influence these psychological states. These states are illustrated in Figure 15.1, a model my associates and I have used many times to stimulate one-on-one and group conversations among employees. We talk of specific situations, operations, or incidents that

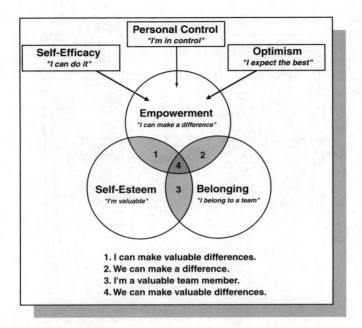

Figure 15.1 Certain person states influence on an individual's willingness to actively care for the safety and health of others.

influence their willingness to actively care for the achievement of a Total Safety Culture. Let's examine these influential states in more detail.

Self-esteem ("I am valuable"). How do you feel about yourself? Generally good or generally bad? Your level of self-esteem is determined by the extent to which you generally feel good about yourself. If we do not feel good about ourselves, it's unlikely we will care about making a difference in the lives of others. As illustrated in Figure 15.2, a person's self-esteem can get pretty low. The better we feel about ourselves, the more willing we are to actively care for the safety and health of other people.

It's important to maintain a healthy level of self-esteem and to help others raise their self-esteem. Research shows that people with high self-esteem report fewer negative emotions and less depression than people with low self-esteem. Those with higher self-esteem also handle life's stresses better. Recall the discussion of stress vs. distress in Chapter 6. Higher self-esteem turns stress into something positive, rather than negative distress.

Researchers have also found that individuals who score higher on measures of self-esteem are less susceptible to outside influences, more confident of achieving personal goals, and make more favorable impressions on others in social situations. And, supporting the actively caring model depicted in Figure 15.1, people with higher self-esteem help others more frequently than those scoring lower on a self-esteem scale.

Empowerment ("I can make a difference"). In the management literature, empowerment typically refers to delegating authority or responsibility, or sharing decision making. In contrast, the person-based perspective of empowerment focuses on how the person who receives more power or influence reacts. From a psychological

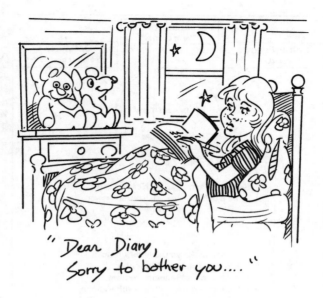

"Dear Diary, Sorry to bother you...."

Figure 15.2 A person's self-esteem can get pretty low.

perspective, empowerment is a matter of personal perception. Do you feel empowered or more responsible? Can you handle the additional assignment? This view of empowerment requires the belief that "I can make a difference."

Perceptions of personal control, self-efficacy, and optimism strengthen the perception of empowerment. An empowered state is presumed to increase motivation to "make a difference," perhaps by going beyond the call of duty. Let's look more closely at these three factors affecting our sense of worth and ability — and our propensity to actively care.

Self-efficacy is the belief that "I can do it." This is a key factor in social learning theory, determining whether a therapeutic intervention will succeed over the long term. We are talking about your self-confidence. Dozens of studies have found that subjects who score relatively high on a measure of self-efficacy perform better at a wide range of tasks. They show more commitment to a goal and work harder to pursue it. They demonstrate greater ability and motivation to solve complex problems at work. They have better health and safety habits and they are more apt to handle stressors positively, rather than with negative distress.

Self-efficacy contributes to self-esteem, and vice versa, but these constructs are different. Simply put, self-esteem refers to a general sense of self-worth; self-efficacy refers to feeling successful or effective at a particular task. Self-efficacy is more focused and can vary markedly from one task to another. One's level of self-esteem remains rather constant across situations.

When I'm losing to an opponent on the tennis court, my self-efficacy usually drops considerably. However, my self-esteem might not change at all. I might protect my self-esteem by rationalizing that my opponent is younger and more experienced or that I'm more physically tired and mentally preoccupied than usual. My damaged self-efficacy will undoubtedly lead to reduced optimism about winning the match. If I continue to lose at tennis and run out of excuses, my self-esteem could suffer *if* I think it is important for me to play tennis well. In this case, there would be a prominent gap between my real self, a loser at tennis, and ideal self, a winner on the court.

Personal control is the feeling that "I am in control." Professor J. B. Rotter (1966) used the term *locus of control* to refer to a general outlook regarding the location of forces controlling a person's life — internal or external. Those with an *internal* locus of control believe they usually have direct personal control over significant life events as a result of their knowledge, skill, and abilities. They believe they are captain of their life's ship.

In contrast, persons with an *external* locus of control believe factors like chance, luck, or fate play important roles in their lives. In a sense, externals believe they are victims, or sometimes beneficiaries, of circumstances beyond their direct personal control. As depicted in Figure 15.3, however, there are times when everyone likes to feel their successes resulted from their own efforts.

Optimism is reflected in the statement, "I expect the best." It's the learned expectation that life events, including personal actions, will turn out well. Compared to pessimists, optimists maintain a sense of humor, perceive problems or challenges in a positive light, and plan for a successful future. *They focus on what they can do rather than on how they feel*. As a result, optimists handle stressors constructively and experience positive stress rather than negative distress. Optimists essentially expect to be successful at whatever they do, and so they work harder than pessimists to reach their goals. As a result, optimists are beneficiaries of the self-fulfilling prophecy. Figure 15.4 shows how an optimistic perspective can influence one's attempt to achieve more.

The self-fulfilling prophecy starts with a personal expectation about one's future performance and ends with that expectation coming true because the individual

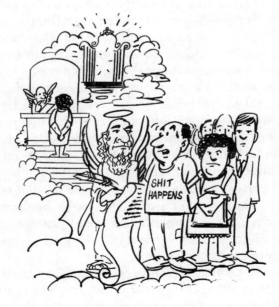

" *Could I take a moment to change my shirt?* "

Figure 15.3 At times, we all want credit for our personal control.

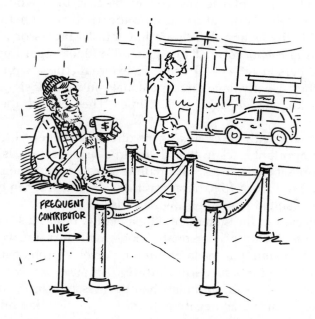

Figure 15.4 Optimists expect more from their efforts.

performs in ways to make it happen. What do you expect when your boss or super-visor asks to see you? Do you expect the best? Our past experiences with top-down control and the use of negative consequences to influence our behavior often result in pessimistic rather than optimistic expectations. Moreover, our approach to this situation, illustrated in Figure 15.5, can support our negative expectations.

If you expect to be punished or reprimanded every time your boss or supervisor calls you into the office, then your body language and demeanor will subtly reflect that expectation. You will "telegraph" these signals to your boss, who might think "Scott sure looks guilty; I wonder what he's done that needs to be punished?"

However, if you approach the interaction with an optimistic attitude, reflected in your body language and verbal behavior, the results could be more positive. You could, for example, write a different internal script. "No one is perfect, and I might have missed something. Everyone can improve with specific behavioral feedback. If I help to make the interaction constructive, the outcome can only be positive."

It's important to understand that fulfilling a pessimistic prophecy can depreciate our perceptions of personal control, self-efficacy, and even self-esteem. Realizing this should motivate us to do whatever we can to make interpersonal conversations positive and constructive. This will not only increase optimism in a work culture but also promote a sense of group cohesiveness or belonging — another person state that facilitates actively caring behavior.

Belonging. In his best seller, *The Different Drum: Community Making and Peace*, Dr. M. Scott Peck (1979) challenges us to experience a sense of true community with others. We need to develop feelings of belonging with one another regardless of our political preferences, cultural backgrounds, and religious doctrine. We need to transcend our differences, overcome our defenses and prejudices, and develop a deep respect for diversity. Peck claims we must develop a sense of community or

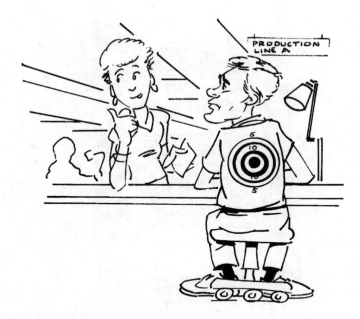

Figure 15.5 When our boss asks to see us, we expect the worse.

interconnectedness with one another if we are to accomplish our best and ensure our survival as human beings. As illustrated in Figure 15.6, the opposite of this perspective or win–lose independence is often experienced on the road, fueling "road rage," and contributing to numerous vehicle crashes and fatalities.

It seems intuitive that building a sense of community or belonging among our coworkers will improve organizational safety. Safety improvement requires interpersonal observation and feedback and, for this to happen, people need to adopt a collective win–win perspective instead of the individualistic win–lose orientation common in many work settings. A sense of belonging and interdependency leads to interpersonal trust and caring — essential features of a Total Safety Culture.

In my numerous group discussions with employees on the belonging concept, someone inevitably raises the point that a sense of belonging or community at their plant has decreased over recent years. "We used to be more like family around here" is a common theme. For many companies, growth spurts, continuous turnover — particularly among managers — or "lean and mean" cutbacks have left many employees feeling less connected and trusting. Figure 15.7 lists a number of special attributes prevalent in most families where interpersonal trust and belonging are often optimal. We are willing to actively care in special ways for the members of our immediate family. The result is optimal trust, belonging, and actively caring behavior for the safety and health of our family members. To the extent we follow the guidelines in Figure 15.7 among members of our "corporate family," we will achieve a Total Safety Culture. Following the principles in Figure 15.7 will develop trust and belonging among people and lead to increasing the quantity and quality of actively caring behavior expected among family members — at home and at work.

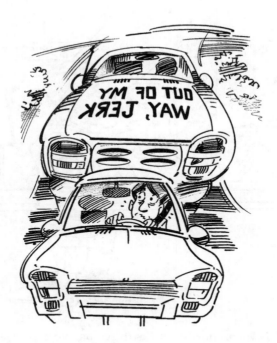

Figure 15.6 A win–lose independent perspective makes vehicle travel more risky.

Actively caring and emotional intelligence

The same person states I have described here as influencing people's willingness to actively care for the safety and health of others also reflect a most important kind of human wisdom — emotional intelligence. How important is emotional intelligence? Well, it's probably much more responsible for our successes and failures in life than mental capacity, or the "intelligence quotient" (IQ) measured by standard IQ tests. From his comprehensive review of the research, Dr. Daniel Goleman (1995) concludes that, "At best, IQ contributes about 20 percent to factors that determine life success, which leaves 80 percent to other factors" (page 34).

Goleman shows convincing evidence that a majority of the other factors contributing to personal achievement can be associated with "emotional intelligence" or one's ability to:

- Remain in control and optimistic following personal failure and frustration; and
- Understand and empathize with other people and work with them cooperatively.

In his influential book, Gardner (1993) refers to the first ability as "intrapersonal intelligence" and the second as "interpersonal intelligence." We show intrapersonal intelligence when we keep our negative emotions (including frustration, anger, sadness, fear, disgust, and shame) in check and use our positive emotions or moods (such as joy, passion, love, optimism, and surprise) to motivate constructive action. The

We use more rewards than penalties with *family* members.

We don't pick on the mistakes of *family* members.

We don't rank one *family* member against another.

We brag on the accomplishments of *family* members.

We respect the property and personal space of *family* members.

We pick up after other *family* members.

We correct the at-risk behavior of *family* members.

We accept the corrective feedback of *family* members.

We are our brothers/sisters keepers of *family* members.

We actively care because they're *family*.

Figure 15.7 Incorporating an actively caring *family* perspective in an organization helps to cultivate a Total Safety Culture.

driver in Figure 15.8 is attempting to control his negative emotions elicited by an unfriendly interpersonal communication.

I'm sure you can see the strong connection between the emotional intelligence concept and the actively caring model discussed previously. Each of the actively caring person states — self-esteem, self-efficacy, personal control, optimism, and belonging — reflects an aspect of emotional intelligence, as conceptualized by Goleman (1995, 1998).

Consider also that actively caring for safety increases emotional intelligence in ourselves and in others. In other words, when we help people avoid taking a calculated risk in order to achieve a delayed and remote positive consequence (avoiding an injury), we increase this special intelligence in ourselves. When these people willingly follow our safety advice and give up the efficiency, comfort, or convenience of an at-risk short cut, they are enhancing this sort of intelligence in themselves.

Safety, emotions, and impulse control

Safety leaders need to develop emotional intelligence in themselves and others. Think about the range of emotions that come into play as we struggle to improve workplace safety and health. We need the curiosity to assess objectively the impact of our safety interventions, persistence to continue successful programs in the face of active resistance, flexibility to try new approaches, resilience to bounce back after failure, and passion to try again.

Achieving the vision of an injury-free workplace requires awareness and control of our own emotions, as well as the ability to assess, understand, and draw on the

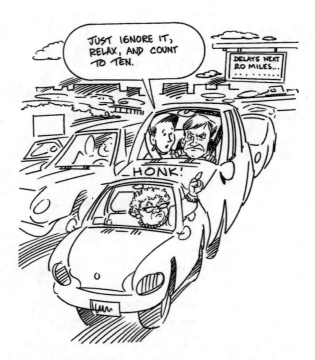

Figure 15.8 Interpersonal communication can affect intrapersonal communication, and vice versa.

influence of other people's emotions. This requires empathic and persuasive communication skills (interpersonal intelligence), as well as self-confidence, personal control, self-esteem, and optimism (intrapersonal intelligence) to develop and implement new tools for safety management.

Perhaps, we can increase personal responsibility for safety by helping people understand the fundamental emotional problem at the root of all safety intervention. Safety requires impulse control under the most difficult circumstances. We ask employees to do things that are uncomfortable or inconvenient in order to avoid a negative consequence that seems remote and improbable. This takes a special kind of emotional intelligence, both from us as safety leaders and from the employees with whom we are working.

Nurturing emotional intelligence

I'm sure you see the relevance of emotional intelligence to improving occupational health and safety. Obviously, safety leaders need to remain self-confident and optimistic (intrapersonal intelligence) in their attempts to prevent injuries, and much of their success depends upon their ability to facilitate involvement, empowerment, and win–win cooperation among those who can be injured (interpersonal intelligence). However, it's easy for safety leaders to get discouraged and frustrated, because so often safety seems to take a back seat to seemingly more immediate demands like meeting production quotas and quality standards.

When we ask people to actively care for health and safety, we're asking them to give up a powerful immediate reward — the ease, speed, or comfort they get from at-risk behavior. In return for extra effort, we promise a bigger reward — they will prevent personal injury or perhaps reduce the possibility a coworker will be injured. Unfortunately, this delayed reward might not seem credible. People have learned they can get away with at-risk behavior, and many people have not made the connection between their own behavior and the reduction of injuries among others.

In conclusion

In this chapter, we continued to develop an understanding of actively caring behavior as it relates to injury prevention. A person-based approach was emphasized; we considered subjective factors inside people as potential determinants of actively caring including their emotional intelligence.

Five person states were proposed as influencing people's willingness to actively care — self-esteem, self-efficacy, personal control, optimism, and belonging. Each of these person variables has a rich research history in psychology and some of this research relates directly to the actively caring model. Research that tested relationships between person states and actual behavior has generally supported the actively caring model.

A particularly important question is whether actively caring states are both antecedents and consequences of a caring act. It seems intuitive that performing an act of kindness that is effective, accepted, and appreciated could increase a helper's self-esteem, self-efficacy, personal control, optimism, and sense of belonging. This, in turn, should increase the probability of more actively caring behavior. In other words, one act of caring, properly appreciated, should lead to another . . . and another. A self-supporting actively caring cycle is likely to occur.

The increasingly popular and research-supported concept of emotional intelligence relates directly to the actively caring model and to improving safety at work, at home, and on the road. Each of the person states in the Actively Caring Model reflects emotional intelligence, and when people go beyond the call of duty to actively care for the safety or health of others, they build emotional intelligence in themselves and in the people they help. Thus, you can see how important it is to get actively caring behavior started and accepted among a large group of individuals. This challenge is addressed in the next chapter.

chapter sixteen

Increasing actively caring behaviors

This chapter integrates principles and procedures from previous chapters to address the most critical question regarding the achievement of a Total Safety Culture. Namely, how can we increase actively caring behavior throughout a work culture? Some conditions and interpersonal techniques facilitate this behavior indirectly by benefiting self-esteem, empowerment, or a sense of belonging. Other procedures can boost actively caring directly with certain activators and consequences. In addition, the social influence principles of reciprocity and consistency can be applied to enhance the caring behavior we desire. In sum, this chapter shows you how to increase the likelihood that people will go beyond their normal routines to help keep people safe.

"In a Total Safety Culture . . . people 'actively care' on a continuous basis for safety."

This quote from my 1994 article in *Professional Safety* (Geller, 1994, page 18) reflects the ultimate vision of a Total Safety Culture. Everyone periodically goes beyond his or her personal routine for the safety and health of others. To meet this challenge, we need to find ways to increase actively caring behaviors.

So how do we do this at work, in our homes, and the community at large? I hope you can already provide some answers after reading Chapters 14 and 15, where I alluded to some ways to increase actively caring behaviors. Here, I want to expand on earlier suggestions and add more. We can classify these approaches as indirect or direct.

Indirect strategies for facilitating actively caring behavior follow from the theory and principles discussed in Chapter 15. The actively caring model supported by research proposes that certain person states inside people increase their willingness to look beyond self-interests and consider the safety of others. Thus, conditions and procedures that increase these states will indirectly increase the amount of actively caring among people. More direct ways to increase these behaviors can be derived from behavior-based principles of learning and social influence. These are discussed in the latter part of this chapter.

Enhancing the actively caring person states

Sometimes at seminars and workshops, I hear participants express concern that the actively caring person-state model might not be practical. "The concepts are too soft or subjective" is a typical reaction. Employees accept the behavior-based approach because it's straightforward, objective, and clearly applicable to the workplace. However, person-based concepts like self-esteem, empowerment, and belonging appear ambiguous, "touchy-feely," and difficult to deal with. "The concepts sound good and certainly seem important, but how can we get our arms around these 'warm fuzzies' and use them to promote safety?"

These person states are more difficult to define, measure, and manage than behaviors. That's why I said early on in this text that it's more cost effective to work on behaviors first. Whenever the ultimate outcome is behavior change, it's usually most efficient to deal directly with behaviors. However, it's always important to consider people's feelings when designing behavior-change interventions. That's why I recommend against using negative consequences whenever possible, and why I offer ways to design intervention strategies that account for subjective person-states like commitment, ownership, and involvement.

After introducing the actively caring person-state model at my workshops, I often divide participants into discussion groups. I ask group members to define events, situations, or contingencies that decrease and increase the person state assigned to their group. Then, I ask the groups to derive simple and feasible action plans to increase their assigned state. This promotes personal and practical understanding of the concept. Let's take a look at what my workshop participants have come up with regarding each of these person states.

Self-esteem

Factors consistently mentioned as shaping self-esteem include communication techniques, reinforcement and punishment contingencies, and leadership styles. Participants suggest a number of ways to build self-esteem, including:

1. Provide opportunities for personal learning and peer mentoring.
2. Increase recognition for desirable behaviors and individual accomplishments.
3. Solicit and follow up on a person's suggestions.

Communication strategies. Figure 16.1 lists 11 words beginning with the letter "A" that imply a specific verbal technique for increasing a person's self-esteem. Each "A" word suggests a slightly different communication approach, from stating simple words of agreement, admiration, appreciation, and approval to acknowledging the achievement and individual creativity of others through active listening and praise. It's also a good idea to argue less and avoid criticizing. Arguments waste time and usually promote a win–lose perspective, and criticism always does more harm than good.

When offering corrective feedback, it's critical to be a patient, active listener. Allow the person to make excuses, and do not argue about these. Resist the temptation. Giving excuses is just a way to protect self-esteem, and it's generally a healthy response. Remember, you already made your point by showing the error and suggesting ways

> • ***Accept*** - appreciate diversity
> • ***Actively Listen*** - with verbal and nonverbal behavior
> • ***Agree*** - with verbal and nonverbal behavior
> • ***Admire*** - "attractive dress," "nice tie"
> • ***Appreciate*** - "please " (activator) and "thank you"
>   (consequence)
> • ***Acknowledge*** - the achievements of other
> • ***Approve*** - praise for good behavior
> • ***Ask*** - for feedback, advice, opinions, etc.
> • ***Attend*** - lend a helping hand
> • ***Avoid Criticizing*** - it won't be accepted anyway
> • ***Argue Less*** - arguments are win/lose situations

Figure 16.1 Apply "A" strategies to increase others' self-esteem.

to avoid the mistake in the future (as discussed in Chapter 12 on coaching). Leave it at that.

Self-efficacy

As I discussed in Chapter 15, self-efficacy is more situation specific than self-esteem, and so it fluctuates more readily. Job-specific feedback should actually affect only one's perception of what is needed to complete a particular task successfully. It should not influence feelings of general self-worth. Keep in mind, though, that repeated negative feedback can have a cumulative effect, chipping away at an individual's self-worth.

Achievable tasks. What makes for a "can do" attitude? Personal perception is the key. A supervisor, parent, or teacher might believe he or she has provided everything needed to complete a task successfully. However, the employee, child, or student might not think so. Hence, the importance of asking, "Do you have what you need?" We are checking for feelings of self-efficacy. This is easier said than done because people often hesitate to admit they are incompetent. Really, who likes to say, "I can't do it?" Instead, we try to maintain the appearance of self-efficacy.

Figure 16.2 reflects the need to focus on "small wins" when assigning tasks and communicating performance feedback. Of course, the kind of situation depicted in Figure 16.2 requires one-on-one observation and feedback in which the individual's initial competencies can be assessed. Then, successively more difficult performance steps can be designed for the learner. The key is to reduce the probability the learner will make an error and feel lowered effectiveness or self-efficacy. Celebrating small-win accomplishments builds self-efficacy and enables support from the self-fulfilling prophecy.

Focus on the positive. Many of the strategies I have presented for improving behaviors and person-states include a basic principle — focus on the positive. Whether attempting to build our own self-efficacy or that of others, success

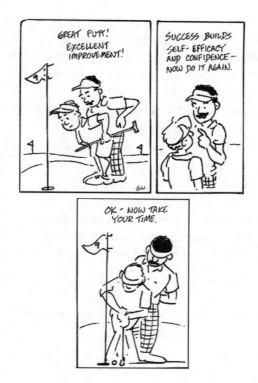

Figure 16.2 Small, successive steps to success build self-efficacy.

needs to be emphasized over failure. Thus, whenever we have the opportunity to teach others or give them feedback, we must look for small-win accomplishments and give genuine approval before commenting on ways to improve. This approach is easier said than done.

Failures are easier to spot than successes. They stick out and disrupt the flow. That's why most teachers give rather consistent negative attention to students who disrupt the classroom, while giving only limited positive attention to students who remain on task and go with the flow. However, considering the impact consequences have on internal person states (especially self-efficacy and self-esteem), a positive consequence (like praise and social approval) is always preferable to a negative consequence (like criticism and ridicule).

Personal control

Employees at my seminars on actively caring have listed a number of ways to increase perceptions of personal control, including:

1. Setting short-term goals and tracking progress toward long-term accomplishment
2. Offering frequent rewarding and correcting feedback for process activities rather than only for outcomes

3. Providing opportunities to set personal goals, teach others, and chart "small wins"
4. Teaching employees basic behavior-change intervention strategies (especially feedback and recognition procedures)
5. Providing people time and resources to develop, implement, and evaluate intervention programs
6. Showing employees how to graph daily records of baseline, intervention, and follow-up data
7. Posting response feedback graphs of group performance

Figure 16.3 illustrates humorously a personal control perspective. Obviously, this is an extreme and unrealistic scenario, but wouldn't it be nice if people would attempt to take personal control of safety issues at their industrial sites with the same passion and commitment some individuals have for their golf game? I believe differences in perceived personal control for safety vs. golf are largely due to contrasting scoring procedures.

Suppose you could not receive direct and immediate feedback about your golf game. That is, each time you hit a golf ball you wore a blindfold and could not see where the ball landed. Even when putting on the greens, you are blindfolded and cannot tell whether your ball goes into the cup. Imagine also that you do not receive a score per hole or per game. However, you do receive negative feedback whenever your ball lands in a sandtrap. Under these circumstances, would you feel "in control" of your golf game? Would you attribute balls hit into sandtraps to personal control or just bad luck? Would you continue playing golf or give it up for an activity in which you can experience greater personal control?

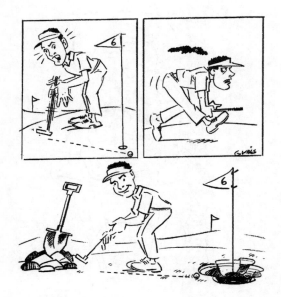

Figure 16.3   Sometimes we try extra hard to exert personal control.

Of course, the golf scenario I asked you to imagine is far-fetched, but is this not the way it is for safety at many industrial sites? The primary evaluation tool used to rank companies and determine performance appraisals and bonuses is an outcome number (such as total recordable injury rate) which is quite remote from the daily plant processes people have control over. Without a scoring system that focuses on controllable processes (as discussed earlier in this book), safety will be viewed as beyond personal control. An injury is just "bad luck," analogous to hitting a golf ball in a sandtrap while blindfolded.

Obviously, we cannot have complete control over all factors contributing to an injury. That's why I think it's wrong to say "*all* injuries are preventable." However, there is much we can do within our own domain of influence, and we can prepare for factors outside our personal control. Thus, we take an umbrella to the golf course in case it rains, and we wear personal protective equipment in case we are exposed to risks beyond our domain of personal control. Likewise, we protect our children from events beyond their control, as illustrated in Figure 16.4.

Optimism

As discussed in Chapter 15, optimism results from thinking positively, avoiding negative thoughts, and expecting the best to happen. Anything that increases our self-efficacy should increase optimism. Also, if our personal control is strengthened, we perceive more influence over our consequences. This gives us more reason to expect the best. Again, we see how the person states of self-efficacy, personal control, and optimism are clearly intertwined. A change in one will likely influence the other two.

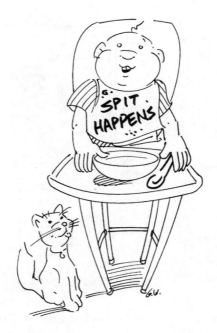

Figure 16.4 We cannot control everything.

Simple events like finding a dime in a coin return, receiving a cookie, listening to soothing music, and being on a winning football team are sufficient to boost optimism and willingness to actively care. It's not necessary for a person to perceive personal control over a pleasant consequence for that consequence to build optimism and possible actively caring behavior.

Belonging

Here are some common proposals given by my seminar discussion groups for creating and sustaining an atmosphere of belonging among employees:

- Decrease the frequency of top-down directives and "quick-fix" programs.
- Increase team-building discussions, group goal-setting and feedback, as well as group celebrations for both process and outcome achievements.
- Use self-managed or self-directed work teams.

When groups are given control over important matters like developing a safety observation and feedback process or a behavior-based incentive program, feelings of both empowerment and belonging can be enhanced. When resources, opportunities, and talents enable team members to assert, "We can make a difference," feelings of belonging occur naturally. This leads to synergy, with the group achieving more than could be possible from members working independently (see Figure 16.5).

Figure 16.6 depicts an obstacle to win–win synergy that I come across all too often. The "we–they" attitude spun off by traditional management–labor differences often makes for dysfunctional work groups. It seems some unions attempt to justify their existence by focusing on disagreement, conflict, and mistrust between management

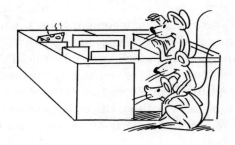

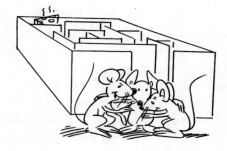

Figure 16.5 Higher goals can be reached through synergy.

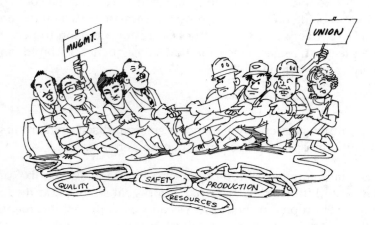

Figure 16.6 Win–lose competition can inhibit teamwork and synergy.

and labor. For its part, management supports this "we–they" split with an alienating communications style that asserts its ultimate power and control. I've seen management memos, for example, that might have been well-intentioned, but were written in top-down, control language that sounded like an adult talking to a child.

Through actively caring, and enhancing self-esteem, empowerment, and belonging, we can bring down the "us vs. them" walls that entrap a work culture. Active caring spreads mutual trust and interdependence throughout the culture. In a Total Safety Culture, everyone benefits from each individual's efforts.

Does actively caring imply the elimination of unions? No, but it might suggest altered visions and mission statements for organized labor groups. Labor unions can certainly help enhance the five person states that facilitate actively caring behavior. To do this, they need to work with management from a win–win perspective that appreciates interdependence and the power of synergy.

At the same time, managers need to relinquish their hold on the "control buttons" of operations and processes that workers can manage themselves, perhaps through self-directed work teams. A truly "empowered work force" is one trusted by managers and supervisors to get the job done without direct supervision. Obviously, this cannot happen overnight, but a solid foundation is cemented when the five actively caring person states are strengthened.

Directly increasing actively caring behaviors

You can treat actively caring behavior just like any other target behavior. Many interventions that increase the occurrence of safe work behaviors can be used to boost the frequency of actively caring behaviors. The four chapters in Part 4 covered principles and procedures for directly influencing behavior. You will recall that the techniques were classified as activators and consequences, with activators considered directive or instructional, and consequences being motivational. Let's take up that discussion again because it applies to actively caring behavior.

Education and training

There's some evidence that educating people about the barriers inhibiting actively caring behavior will increase acts of caring. The impact of education should be even more dramatic if some of the concepts discussed in Chapter 14 are taught. It seems particularly useful to explain that actively caring behavior can be proactive or reactive, direct or indirect, and focused on the environment, internal person states, or behavior. Also, it should be taught that direct, proactive, and behavior-focused active caring is most challenging — and most useful to prevent injuries.

Consequences for actively caring

Rewards should increase actively caring behavior. This comes from the basic operant learning principle that behavior increases following positive consequences. But it's perhaps even more important not to respond negatively when observing a caring act. A negative reaction could make that person avoid a subsequent opportunity to actively care for safety. I made a similar point when discussing safety coaching in Chapter 12. A person's reaction to a safety coach could determine whether or not that person goes out of his or her way to coach again for safety.

The "actively caring thank-you cards" described in Chapter 11 are a rather generic technique to boost caring in the workplace. You will recall that employees used these cards to thank their colleagues for going beyond the call of duty for the safety of others. Some cards included a space for the intervention agent to define the act of caring. Some cards could be exchanged for inexpensive rewards, like a beverage in the company cafeteria. Other cards had peel-off stickers for public display. In some applications, each card was worth some amount of money (e.g., $1.00) toward corporate contributions to local charities.

The reciprocity principle

Some sociologists, anthropologists, and moral philosophers consider reciprocity a universal norm that motivates a good deal of interpersonal behavior. Simply put, people are expected to help those who have helped them. You can expect people to comply with your request if you have done a favor for them. This is the principle behind Stephen Covey's (1989) claim that we need to make deposits in another person's emotional bank account before making a withdrawal.

Have you ever felt a little uncomfortable after someone did you a favor? I certainly have. I interpret my discomfort as the reciprocity principle in action. Another person's kind act makes me feel pressured to respond in kind. What does this mean for safety? I think it means we should look for opportunities to go out of our way for another person's safety. Doing this, we increase the likelihood they will help when we need them.

Gifts aren't free. Has someone snared your attention to hear a sales pitch after giving you a free gift? Have you ever felt obligated to contribute to a charity after receiving gummed individualized address labels and a stamped envelope for your check? Ever purchase food in a supermarket after eating a free sample? Do you feel obliged to buy something after using it for a ten-day "free" trial period?

If you answer "yes" to any of these questions, it's likely you have been influenced by the reciprocity principle. Many marketing or sales-promotion efforts count on this "free sample" gimmick to influence purchasing behavior. Does this justify distributing free safety gifts, such as pens, tee-shirts, caps, cups, and other trinkets? Yes, to some extent, but you have to take into account perceptions. How special is the gift? Was the gift given to a select group of people, or was it distributed to everyone? Does the gift or its delivery represent significant sacrifice in money, time, or effort? Can it be purchased elsewhere, or does its safety slogan make it special?

A "special" safety gift — as perceived by the recipient — will trigger more acts of caring in response. Remember, too, that the way a gift is bestowed can make all the difference in the world. The labels and slogans linked with it can influence the amount and kind of responsive action. If the gift is presented to represent the actively caring safety leadership expected from a "special" group of workers, a certain type of reciprocity is activated. People will tell themselves they are considered leaders, and they need to justify this label by going beyond the call of duty for others. If they have learned about the various categories of actively caring behavior, they know the best way to lead is by taking action that is direct, proactive, and focused on supporting safe behavior or correcting at-risk behavior.

Commitment and consistency

Robert Cialdini refers to commitment and consistency as an influence mechanism lying deep within us, directing many of our actions. It reflects our motivation to be, and appear to be, consistent. "Once we make a choice or take a stand, we will encounter personal and interpersonal pressures to behave consistently with that commitment" (Cialdini, 2001, page 53). Cialdini suggests the pressure comes from three basic sources:

- Society values consistency within people.
- Consistent conduct benefits daily existence.
- A consistent orientation allows us to take shortcuts when processing information and making decisions. We do not have to stop to consider everything involved; instead we fall back on our prior commitment or decision and act accordingly to remain true to ourselves.

Public and voluntary commitment. The "safe behavior promise card" described in Chapter 10 derives its power to influence from the commitment and consistency principle. When people sign their name to a promise card they commit to behaving in a certain way. Then, they act in a way that is consistent with their commitment.

Commitments are most effective, or influential, when they are visible, require some amount of effort, and are perceived to be voluntary, not coerced. It makes sense, then, to have employees state a public rather than private commitment to actively care for safety and to have them sign their names to a promise card rather than merely raising their hands. It's critically important for those making a pledge to believe they did it voluntarily. In reality, decisions to make a public commitment are dramatically influenced by external activators and consequences, including peer pressure. However, if people sell themselves on the idea that they made a personal choice, consistency is likely to follow the commitment.

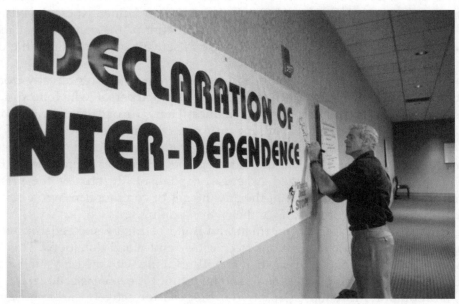

Figure 16.7 The author signs a "Declaration of Interdependence."

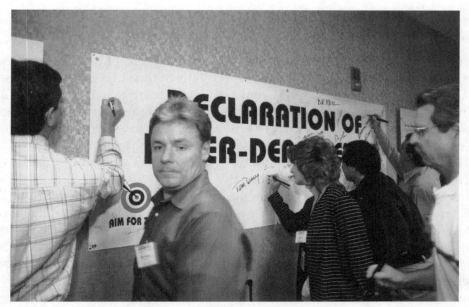

Figure 16.8 Delta Airlines employees sign a "Declaration of Interdependence."

Figures 16.7 and 16.8 illustrate a public commitment intervention implemented at a safety seminar for supervisors, safety leaders, and maintenance personnel of Delta Airlines. After giving a keynote address on the concept of actively caring for the safety and health of others, I signed my name to a "Declaration of Interdependence" as a symbol of commitment to look out for the safety of others (Figure 16.7). Then, I urged the audience to follow suit.

The social context was partly responsible for the great number of individuals signing the declaration (Figure 16.8) which is now prominently displayed at the employees' worksite. The public and voluntary nature of the commitment request contributed to the effectiveness of this exercise to activate awareness and the development of relevant action plans.

Foot-in-the-door: Start small and build. This strategy follows directly from the commitment and consistency principle. To be consistent, a person who follows a small request will likely comply with a larger request later. During the Korean War, the Chinese communists used this technique on American prisoners by gradually escalating their demands, which started with a few harmless requests. First, prisoners were persuaded to speak or write trivial statements. Then they were urged to copy or create statements that criticized American capitalism. Eventually, the prisoners participated in group discussions of the advantages of communism, wrote self-criticisms, and gave public confessions of their wrong-doing.

Research has found this "start small and build" strategy succeeds in boosting product sales, monetary contributions to charities, and blood donations. This "foot-in-the-door" technique only works when people go along with the first small request. If a person says "No" right away, he or she might find it even easier to resist subsequent, more important requests. So, if your first call for actively caring behavior is shot down, you did not start small enough. Be prepared to retreat to something less demanding and build reciprocity from there.

In conclusion

The information reviewed in this chapter is critical in terms of practical application. Integrating principles and procedures from prior chapters, I've tried to address this crucial challenge. Continuous safety improvement leading to a Total Safety Culture requires people to actively care – for others as well as themselves. Research-derived procedures to increase the frequency of actively caring behavior throughout a culture were discussed. Some of these influence techniques indirectly increase actively caring behavior by benefiting the person states that facilitate one's willingness to care. Other influence strategies target behaviors directly.

Indirect strategies are deduced from the actively caring model explained in Chapter 15. Any procedure that increases a person's self-esteem, perception of empowerment — including self-efficacy, personal control, and optimism — or sense of belonging or group cohesion will indirectly benefit active caring. A number of communication techniques enhance more than one of these states simultaneously, in particular actively listening to others for feelings and giving genuine praise for accomplishments. There are barriers to focusing on the positive, and we discussed these in the hope that awareness will help overcome the obstacles.

The behavior-change techniques detailed in Part 4 of this text — from setting SMART goals and signing promise cards to offering soon, certain, and positive consequences for the right behavior — can be used to enhance those actively caring person states. They can also directly increase actively caring behavior. Education and direct participation in actively caring projects foster the behavior we are seeking as well.

The interpersonal influence principles of reciprocity and consistency were introduced as they apply to our everyday decisions and behaviors. The consistency principle is behind the success of safe behavior promise cards, and the foot-in-the-door technique ("start small and build"). These principles and specific strategies can be applied to directly boost actively caring behaviors.

part six

Putting it all together

chapter seventeen

Promoting high-performance teamwork

Everyone talks about teamwork, but not everyone gets the best from their teams. Teamwork just does not come naturally. This chapter explains why and what we can do about it. Principles and practical procedures are offered for initiating and sustaining productive teamwork. The functions of seven different safety teams are described. Each of these teams contributes to improving the human dynamics of occupational safety, as taught in this book. Each team depends on the output of other teams to optimize the system and cultivate a Total Safety Culture.

"My responsibility is to get my 25 guys playing for the name on the front
of their uniform and not the name on the back." — Tommy Lasorda

Imagine a workplace where everyone coaches each other about the safest way to perform a job. A workplace in which actively caring for other people's safety is a natural part of the everyday routine. When people depend on each other in this way to improve safety, they understand teamwork. They have an interdependent mindset and realize the true meaning of synergy. For these individuals TEAM means Together Everyone Achieves More.

Reaching this level of teamwork does not come easily. After all, look at how we have been raised. "Be independent," we are told. We compete with other individuals to get ahead, whether at work or at play. Remember, "Nice guys finish last." A win–lose, me-first mindset is promoted by almost everything in our culture, from the grades we get in school to salary promotions at work.

This chapter is about win–win teamwork. It builds on the principles of behavior-based safety presented in Part 3, the intervention tools from behavior-based safety detailed in Part 4, and the concepts of group belonging and interdependence discussed in Part 5.

Cultivating high-performance teamwork

Let's consider the main phases of teamwork, from start to finish, and see how each relates to the development of optimum group performance for safety improvement. Here, I provide real-world answers to questions like "How can we establish a successful safety team?" and "Once we have a safety team, what can we do to make it more effective?"

Figure 17.1 outlines seven consecutive phases of teamwork, from selecting team members to disbanding or renewing the team. These are the basic steps of teamwork as discussed by leading team-building trainers and consultants. Let's examine each of these steps in more detail as they relate specifically to industrial safety.

Selecting team members

Obviously, the first crucial step in successful safety teamwork is to select the right people for your team. Someone is ultimately responsible for choosing team members. In safety, this is often the safety director or the person responsible for maintaining injury reports and lost-time records. In some cases, however, it's advantageous for a small committee of safety champions representing a cross section of the workforce to select *potential* members of a safety team. I say "potential" because it's important for membership to be voluntary. So, a safety champion or selection committee should come up with a list of people to approach one-on-one and ask if they would be willing to serve on a particular safety team.

So, what kinds of people should you look for as potential members of a safety team? Perhaps, first and foremost, the candidate should be committed to safety. Has

1. **Select the Right Team Members**
   - Understand and appreciate behavior-based safety.
   - Commitment, interpersonal interest, communication, and caring.
2. **Clarify the Assignment**
   - State general mission or purpose.
   - Specify resources, authority, and accountability.
   - Get acquainted.
   - Develop understanding of TEAM, interdependency, and synergy.
3. **Establish a Team Charter**
   - Write a mission statement.
   - Set ground rules.
   - Define deliverables and accountability.
   - Specify budget details and direct reports.
   - Assign standard team roles.
4. **Develop Action Plan**
   - Set goals with SMARTS.
   - Assign task responsibilities.
   - Develop time lines.
5. **Engage in the Process**
   - Conduct productive team meetings.
   - Use brainstorming and consensus-building.
   - Give each other supportive and corrective behavior-based feedback.
6. **Evaluate Team Performance**
   - Recognize process results.
   - Document product results.
   - Celebrate accomplishments.
7. **Disband, Restructure, or Renew the Team**

Figure 17.1 Follow seven steps for team success.

the individual done something recently to indicate personal concern for the safety or health of a coworker? Perhaps, she turned in a comprehensive near-hit report in a work culture where such reports are rare or, maybe, the employee was injured recently and has given testimony to a renewed regard for safety initiatives.

Besides demonstrating special commitment to occupational safety, the best team members also have other qualities. They have interpersonal skills (they like to work with other people), they communicate well (they actively listen and speak with passion), and they are willing to actively care for the safety and health of others.

Clarify the assignment

From the start, it's important for the team members to understand their assignment. They need to know the overall mission of the team and the resources available to accomplish it. They also need to understand their authority with regard to the mission. For example, they need to realize the degree of control the team has over the consequences of their decisions. Will any other authority influence the outcome of the team's decisions? In other words, to what extent is the team truly empowered to carry out the processes needed to accomplish its mission?

This is when the true purpose of a team is discussed. Why is the assignment given to a team instead of individuals working alone? What are the advantages of using a team? Own up to the fact that the start-up process will take some time, and some might think one dedicated person would be more efficient. In the long run, however, teamwork will be more effective. Now it's appropriate to explain the TEAM acronym — Together Everyone Achieves More.

Besides explaining the general mission and the TEAM concept, the team facilitator should also provide opportunities for the participants to get acquainted. Introductions could be initiated with a statement like "Let's get to know each other better by each person stating your name, your job, and your general expectations, if any, about our team assignment." Later, you might also ask each team member to say something about safety: "Tell us about your personal interest or commitment to occupational safety."

Establish a team charter

During the prior "getting acquainted" phase, the mission was given as a general description of the team's assignment. Now, it's time to write a formal mission statement that articulates the overall purpose of the team, define the ground rules for team meetings, address budget issues, specify what the team will produce (its deliverables), and assign various team roles. Some standard team roles are as follows, although I have seen many situations where one person assumes more than one role:

- Team leader — provides direction and obtains outside resources.
- Team facilitator — keeps meetings focused and prompts total participation.
- Team administrator — handles various administrative duties like distributing reports, networking with outside individuals and groups, and reminding members of team meetings.
- Treasurer — tracks input and output of finances.
- Reporter — documents and distributes meeting agenda and minutes.

It's vital that each team member understands and affirms the mission statement, deliverables, ground rules, accountability system, and team role assignments. Therefore, a "team charter" is developed through consensus-building, which is the opposite of top-down decision making. It's not the same as negotiating, calling for a vote and letting the majority win, or working out a compromise between two different sets of opinions. The team facilitator in Figure 17.2 is not likely to cultivate consensus.

Building consensus. Negotiating, voting, or compromising comes across as win–lose and decreases the interpersonal trust needed for high performance teamwork. A majority of the team might be pleased, but others will be discontented and might actively or passively resist involvement. Even the "winners" could feel lowered interpersonal trust. "We won this decision, but what about next time?" Without everyone's buy-in for a group decision, the teamwork will be less synergistic than possible.

So how can group consensus be developed? How can the outcome of a heated debate on ways to solve a problem be perceived as a win–win solution everyone supports, instead of a win–lose compromise or negotiation? Practical answers to these questions are easier said than done. Consensus-building takes time, energy, and patience. It requires open and frank conversation among all team members.

The scenario depicted in Figure 17.3 is unacceptable. All participants must be willing to state their honest opinion without fear of ridicule or reprisal. It takes a good team facilitator to make this happen. He or she needs to solicit the opinions of everyone throughout the team meeting.

There's no quick fix to do this. It requires plenty of interpersonal communication, including straightforward opinion sharing, intense discussion, emotional debate, proactive listening, careful evaluation, methodical organization, and systematic prioritizing. On important matters, however, the outcome is well worth the investment. When you develop a solution or process every potential participant can get behind and champion, you have cultivated the degree of interpersonal trust and ownership

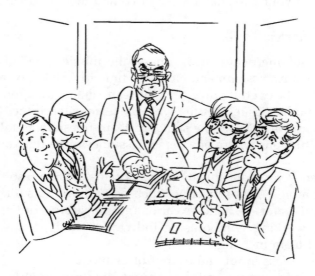

Figure 17.2 Body language speaks louder than words.

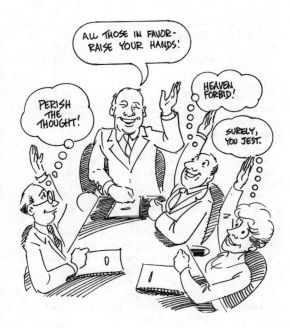

Figure 17.3 Census building requires frank and open communication.

needed for total involvement. Involvement, in turn, builds personal commitment, more ownership, and then more involvement.

Developing ground rules. Total participation of every team member during important discussions is vital for consensus-building. Thus, open and frank discussion should be a team-meeting ground rule accepted by everyone. Figure 17.4 lists this and other potential ground rules to consider adopting for increasing the effectiveness of your team meetings. These are general guidelines or rules of conduct the team members need to agree on and hold each other accountable to follow.

You should not just post the contents of Figure 17.4 and call them "our team ground rules." Rather, you need to discuss the issue of ground rules with team members and get everyone's opinion. Then, use a consensus-building approach to get everyone's acceptance of the final list. You can use the suggestions in Figure 17.4 to "prime the pump" or stimulate discussion, or just keep the seven items in mind as you facilitate group discussion and look for opportunities to direct comments toward these topics.

Writing a mission statement. You can use this basic consensus-building approach to arrive at a mission statement. In other words, you should have a basic idea of the team's overall mission or purpose. Then, use consensus building to write a mission statement everyone can support. Be sure to explain that the team's mission statement must be a clearly stated purpose that serves to direct and motivate team members. It answers three basic questions:

- What does the team do?
- How does the team do its work?
- Who are the team's customers?

1. **Everyone participates**.
   Active participation comes with the territory. This means always being prepared for team meetings and problem-solving discussions.
2. **No barbs or put-downs**.
   Team members show respect for each other. They don't say anything that could hurt someone's feelings or limit the involvement of others.
3. **Every idea counts**.
   Team members listen with respect to everyone's opinion regardless of how silly it might seem at first. The strangest sounding idea can be the seed for creative invention.
4. **Strive to be completely informed**.
   Team members actively listen during team meetings to know exactly what's going on. They openly ask questions about anything they don't fully understand.
5. **Follow through on commitments and meet deadlines**.
   Keeping promises builds interpersonal trust and assures team progress. This includes showing up for *all* meetings on time.
6. **Support team decisions**.
   Team members voice their concerns during decision-making discussions because in the end they realize they must support a team decision.
7. **Think win/win interdependency**.
   Team members want everyone to win. Synergy depends on everyone contributing individual talents for the good of all.

Figure 17.4 Seven ground rules can promote effective team meetings.

Develop an action plan

Keeping in mind the team mission and ground rules, the team now plans how it will proceed. This planning process consists of three primary steps:

- Define specific goals needed to accomplish the mission.
- Decide on a time line for completing each goal.
- Assign goal-relevant tasks to each team member.

Let's consider some general approaches to taking these steps. The specifics will vary depending upon the safety mission, the team charter, and the talents, skills, and opinions of the team members. Remember to follow the basic consensus-building process when arriving at goals and assigning tasks.

Define tasks. Process goals imply specific tasks, while outcome goals do not. For example, the process goal, "complete 100 behavior-based observation sessions by the end of the month" is quite task specific and stipulates what needs to be done. In contrast, the outcome goal "to reduce the total recordable injury rate by 50 percent this year" does not suggest any actions or behaviors. Assuming this outcome goal is judged achievable by the team, it's necessary to decide on specific tasks needed to achieve the goal. One of those tasks might be, in fact, to conduct periodic behavior-based observations throughout a work area. In this case, the process goal to achieve 100 observations would be needed to attain the outcome of reduced injuries.

It would likely take several process goals to reach a certain injury-reduction goal. Process goals could be derived for attendance of safety meeting, for reporting of near hits and property damage incidents, for removing environmental hazards, and for engaging in one-on-one safety-related conversations with coworkers. All of these are tasks that could contribute to reaching an injury-reduction milestone. So, the achievement of an injury-reduction outcome goal is contingent on reaching certain process goals. All of these goals are consistent with the mission or purpose of obtaining an injury-free workplace.

Assign task responsibilities. The key to successful teamwork is to develop a list of specific tasks needed to achieve team goals and, then, to assign the right persons to take on the various task responsibilities. Also critical, of course, is the setting of appropriate deadlines for each task to be completed. Adding a deadline or completion date for specific assignments results in a SMARTS goal. These goals are SMART, as discussed earlier in Chapter 10, with "S" for specific, "M" for motivational, "A" for achievable, "R" for relevant, and "T" for trackable. The added "S" for SMARTS team goals stands for shared. SMARTS goals are then organized into a time line for scheduling teamwork.

Make it happen

After setting SMARTS goals, assigning task responsibilities, and developing a time line, the real work begins. Process goals have been set and team members are motivated to fulfill their interdependent roles for the sake of their team mission. This is the performing stage of teamwork. Regular team meetings are still needed to keep the process going and to promote continuous improvement. More specifically, team meetings provide opportunities for team members to connect with one another and:

- Hold each other accountable for achieving specific tasks.
- Review project progress and acknowledge achievements of individuals, subgroups, and the team as a whole.
- Discuss problems and entertain corrective action plans.
- Check the time line and make refinements and additions.
- Plan for next steps and assign new task responsibilities.

Prepare an agenda. A well-planned and well-run meeting starts with an agenda. This keeps the meeting on track and focused, and prevents off-track or time-wasting behavior. A good agenda is neither wordy nor complex. It's simply an outline of items to be covered.

At the start of the meeting a copy of the agenda should be distributed to all participants. When participants keep an agenda in front of them throughout the meeting, they are apt to keep their comments on track. This also prompts team members to offer their perspectives and recommendations at the appropriate times.

The basic structure of the agenda will not vary much from one meeting to the next. The following components make up most meeting agendas and occur in the order given here.

- Review the purpose of the team meeting.
- Make any organizational announcements relevant to the team's mission.

- Call for progress reports from team members, including project objectives, accomplishments since the last meeting, and special assistance or resources needed for the next steps.
- Discuss special issues, difficulties, and solutions with a focus on the positive or on examining ways to overcome problems raised.
- Identify what needs to happen next per project or task assignment in order to progress and continuously improve.
- Set the time and date for the next meeting and offer a preview of critical topics or project reports to be covered.

Manage time well. How many times have you heard someone say, "I could get so much more done in a day if I didn't have so many meetings to go to"? Meetings have the reputation of robbing people of valuable time. So, if time is managed well at your safety team meetings, everyone will be appreciative. More will get accomplished, and people will feel good about the time they gave up. I suggest the following for managing your meeting time effectively:

- Designate a start and stop time, and make sure everyone knows what these are.
- Start the meeting on time, even if everyone has not shown up. This sets the stage for on-time arrivals.
- Stop the meeting on time, even if every agenda item was not covered completely. This sets the stage for efficient use of meeting time.
- Allot specific time periods to each agenda item and remind participants of these throughout the meeting.
- If breaks are given, state a precise time for participants to return. Start the meeting again at this time, even if everyone has not returned.
- If discussions get long, remind participants of the time remaining and the number of agenda items left.
- Hold meetings prior to lunch time or at the end of the workday in order to provide an incentive to get things done on time.
- Do not allow cellular phones or pagers in the meetings or you will set the stage for distraction.

Record minutes. Decisions and assignments made during a team meeting are usually critical for team success, yet they can be easily forgotten. Therefore, it's important for someone to document key events of the team meeting. When team members are confident the designated "recorder" will take good notes, they will not be distracted by their own note-taking behavior. They can listen attentively and participate actively throughout the meeting. Later the meeting notes are made available as a permanent record of team progress. This reminds teammates of their accomplishments and their obligations for continual success.

Communicate between meetings. Team members need to support each other when completing their assignments. Don't wait until the next team meeting to inquire about a teammate's progress on a project. Asking others how their specific assignments are going sends the message you care about their contributions to your team. Taking the time to listen to a report of progress or actually reviewing results from a particular assignment does more to show your concern and can be a powerful motivator.

It is awfully important to give supportive and corrective feedback for specific behaviors related to team assignments. As I discussed in Chapter 16, behavior-based feedback is extremely powerful in directing and motivating desirable behavior. Team members need to be alert to the kinds of behaviors needed from each other in order to have a successful team. They also need to follow certain guidelines for giving effective feedback to their teammates, as I detailed in Chapter 12.

Evaluate team performance

I'm sure you realize the value of performance evaluation when it's done well. In fact, the discussion in the previous section about feedback says it all. Willing workers cannot improve without receiving feedback directly related to their performance, and such feedback is only available through an objective and periodic evaluation process. Evaluation is the key to accountability and responsibility as I detail in the next chapter. Here, I offer a few guidelines regarding the evaluation of safety teams so they might improve their performance.

My guess is most readers will find Figure 17.5 humorous. Why? What is the problem with most performance appraisals? If performance appraisals were objective, fair, and based on behavior, you would not see any humor in this illustration. Right! So, a useful evaluation of team performance needs to be objective, fair, and related to changeable behaviors and conditions.

Your team needs to evaluate its performance periodically in order to assess successive improvements made possible by prior evaluations. Then, it has reason to celebrate its accomplishments. Quality team celebrations (as discussed in Chapter 13) are key to enhancing team cohesiveness and mutual responsibility toward the accomplishment of more shared goals.

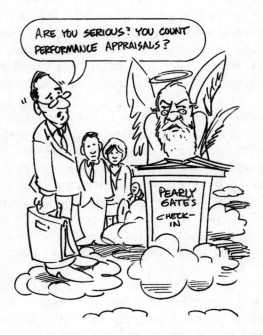

Figure 17.5 Subjective, nonbehavioral, and infrequent evaluations are not taken seriously.

It's important to realize that although performance evaluation is listed sixth in this list of successive teamwork steps, this topic is inherent in every step. Whether selecting team members, establishing a team charter, or setting goals and assigning task responsibilities, evaluation plays an integral role.

Team members continually evaluate each other's opinions and reactions throughout group discussions in order to arrive at decisions everyone can support. The presentation of project reports at team meetings is essentially an evaluation process. Team members appraise whether a project is progressing as planned and decide whether the time line needs adjusting when the results call for refinements or additions to the list of task assignments. All of this involves the ongoing study and interpretation of information in order to make the best decisions. This is evaluation in the truest sense of the word.

Disband, restructure, or renew the team

Many books and manuals on teamwork discuss this final stage as the time when members of a work team realize their work is done and adjourn or disband. This is rarely the case, however, for safety teams. The work of these teams is never done. Consider, for example, the seven teams defined in Figure 17.6 which I propose are needed to address comprehensively the human dynamics of industrial safety.

Specific projects or assignments may come and go, but safety teams need to work persistently on their general missions in order to achieve continuous safety improvement throughout a work culture. The membership of these teams will change periodically and team goals will vary, but the challenges of behavioral observation and feedback, incident analysis and corrective action, ergonomics analysis and intervention, and behavior-based recognition and celebration will remain. Of course, the methods and procedures used to meet these team functions will change and, in fact, they will successfully improve if appropriate evaluation processes are implemented.

Safety teams will learn to work more effectively and efficiently over time, but they will need to keep working. Even when your workplace becomes injury free, the safety teams listed in Figure 17.6 are needed to maintain this enviable situation. Thus, this final step for safety team success should be considered restructuring or renewing, not disbanding.

Restructuring. Restructuring could mean a change in focus, in team membership, or in the methods and procedures the team uses to accomplish its mission. For example, after observation and feedback teams are in operation throughout your work culture, the Safety Steering Team changes its focus from promoting and training to advising and maintaining. In other words, after employee teams get involved in behavior-based coaching, the challenge becomes one of sustaining the process. The prime issue changes from "how we can teach coworkers behavior-based coaching procedures and convince work teams to use critical behavior checklists on a regular basis" to "how we can keep work teams motivated to keep their behavior-based observation and feedback process going."

In the beginning, the efforts of the Incentive/Reward Team might focus on convincing management and coworkers to substitute behavior-based safety incentives for their traditional safety incentive program that offers rewards for reductions in injury rate. If successful at this, the team's challenge changes to developing an

Safety Steering Team — oversees the effort of all other teams listed here.
Observation and Feedback Team — develops, implements, evaluates, and refines behavior-based observation and feedback procedures.
Ergonomics Team — conducts periodic audits of workplace settings, evaluates employee suggestions regarding ergonomic issues, and recommends corrective action for environment, behavior, or both.
Incident Analysis Team — conducts fact-finding evaluations of near-hit reports and injuries, including behavioral, environment, and person-based factors; and recommends corrective action.
Celebration Team — plans and manages celebration events to recognize process activities and reward achievements of milestones.
Incentives/Rewards Team — oversees the design, implementation, evaluation, and refinement of behavior-based incentive/reward programs to motivate participation in designated safety-improvement activities.
Preventive Action Team — evaluates reports of rule/policy violations, decides whether the violator should be punished, and chooses the penalty.

Figure 17.6 Various types of employee teams are needed to improve occupational safety.

acceptable and effective behavior-based safety incentive program. Then, the team needs to evaluate the impact of this incentive program and refine it for another application. This plan–implement–evaluate–refine process needs to be repeated over the long term to maximize the beneficial impact of behavior-based safety incentives.

Earlier in Chapter 11, I presented details on the design, administration, and evaluation of safety incentive programs. My point here is that each of the four key phases — planning, implementing, evaluating, and refining — implies a different team focus, along with unique goals and task assignments. Special training, resources, and individual talents are needed for each phase, requiring appropriate adjustment in team leadership, meeting agenda, and task assignments. These four phases are not peculiar to a Safety Incentive/Reward Team. They are relevant for each of the seven safety teams listed in Figure 17.6.

Nothing helps a team more to stay motivated and aligned with its mission than an objective presentation of the good they have done and an opportunity to learn how to improve their intervention and do more good. This is the essence of an objective and equitable accountability system which leads to people's responsibility for safety extending beyond the numbers. As I detail elsewhere (Geller, 1998a), this is fundamental to attaining and maintaining an injury-free workplace.

Renewing. When team members observe the "fruits" of their labor, their motivation to continue their efforts is bolstered. In other words, observation of success breeds more success. So, an optimal way to renew the confidence and purpose of a team is to display clear and objective evidence that their efforts make a difference. More can and should be done, however, to move teams forward with renewed concern and commitment.

Team-building sessions can be conducted with the sole purpose of restoring team members' motivation toward teamwork. Often, it's beneficial to hire an outside consultant or facilitator to conduct such a session. However, it's possible your company training department employs a person who could facilitate an effective team-building session.

In conclusion

This is, obviously, only a brief overview of basic steps involved in developing and sustaining high-performance safety teams. Additional details related to each of these procedural steps are available in other texts (e.g., Geller, 1998b; Lloyd, 1996; Parker, 1996; Rees, 1997). You realize, of course, that effective safety teams do not develop overnight. Each process reviewed here takes time and patient application of the various interpersonal and group process strategies described in Parts 3 and 4 of this text, including behavior-based observation and feedback, proactive listening, directive and supportive coaching, individual recognition, and actively caring performance evaluations.

The benefits of implementing these teamwork strategies will not be immediate. The "sell" for teamwork is analogous to the "sell" for safety. Safety leaders are well aware of the need to perform certain inconvenient, inefficient, and even uncomfortable safety-related behaviors in order to reap the potential long-term benefits of injury prevention. Likewise, the rewards of teamwork require substantial up-front investment in resources, time, and collective effort.

Many of us are not used to the collaborative and cooperative interdependency of high-performance teamwork. This includes the people who hold us accountable for our work output. Therefore, the teamwork perspective of mutual accountability for shared goals needs to be appreciated by managers and supervisors as well as by team members. The people in organizations who provide the resources and opportunities for teamwork need to understand what it takes to reap the benefits of synergy, even if they are not members of a team themselves.

Figure 17.7 depicts a typical scenario in the hustle and bustle of our everyday lives. Everyone is doing his or her own thing from a win–lose, individualistic framework. The outcome seems like utter chaos and leaves individuals with the impression that their personal goals are temporarily thwarted. This can lead to frustration and a bad attitude toward the whole situation. A bad attitude can influence risky or win–lose behavior, which in turn adds fuel to a bad attitude.

Our hero in Figure 17.7 has a different perspective on the whole situation. He is able to take a broader view and appreciate the marvelous interdependent transportation system. This viewpoint, or systems-thinking paradigm, toward everyday circumstances can be greatly beneficial to the safety and health of individuals and groups.

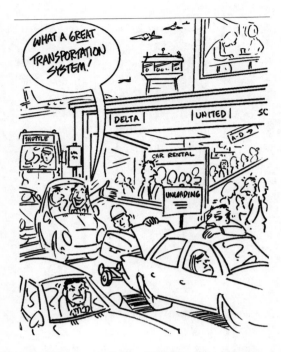

Figure 17.7 Systems thinking reflects the interdependency paradigm needed for high-performance teamwork.

Systems thinking benefits teamwork *and* it is a consequence of teamwork. Therefore, systems thinking feeds the interdependency and collectiveness needed for high-performance teams, and productive teamwork feeds more systems thinking. This attitude-behavior spiral is constructive and motivates the special commitment and dedication needed to build and maintain successful safety teams.

chapter eighteen

Evaluating for continuous improvement

Continuous improvement demands proper evaluation. This chapter explains how to evaluate the impact of safety interventions from an environment, behavior, and person perspective. More employees need to contribute information pertinent to intervention evaluation. This chapter shows you how to make this happen. The principles described here will make you a smarter consumer of marketed safety programs and help you evaluate your own customized intervention process.

"What gets measured gets done; what gets measured and rewarded gets done well." — Larry Hansen

Larry Hansen (1994) used these words in his *Professional Safety* article on managing occupational safety (page 41). You have probably heard words to this effect. Indeed, they're key to any continuous improvement effort. But there's a problem with how workplace safety is traditionally measured. As I indicated in Chapter 3, too much weight is given to outcome numbers people cannot control directly. People must be held accountable for results they *can* control. Yet, corporations, divisions, plants, and departments are often ranked according to abstract outcome numbers like the total recordable injury rate. These rankings often determine bonus rewards or penalties.

What behavior improves when safety awards are based only on an injury rate? If employees can link their daily activities to safety results, then celebrating reduced injury rates can be useful, even motivating. It's critical, however, to recognize the behaviors, procedures, and processes that led to fewer injuries or lower workers' compensation costs.

If you don't focus on the real causes of improvement, you run the risk of actually demotivating the folks deserving recognition. Employees might think continuous improvement is caused by luck or chance — events beyond personal control. This can lead to feelings of apathy or perceived helplessness as I discussed earlier (e.g., see Chapters 6, 15, and 16). If we want employees to work for continuous improvement, we need to recognize and reward the "right stuff." This requires the right kind of measurement procedures.

Measuring the right stuff

Deming (1991) admonished his audiences for ranking people, departments, and organizations. In fact, he recommended that grades and performance appraisals be abolished completely from education and business. In his words, "The fact is that performance appraisal, management by the numbers, M.B.O., and work standards have already devastated Western industry . . . the annual rating of performance has devastated Western industry . . . Western management has for too long focused on the end product" (Deming, 1986a, page 1).

Part of Deming's rationale comes from the fact that standard approaches to measuring academic and work performance are often subjective, relative, and not clearly related to individual behavior. Teachers and professors, for example, use contrived distribution curves and cut-offs to assure only a designated percentage of students can attain certain grades. Knowledge tests are necessarily biased and imperfect assessment devices, and are often only remotely linked to specific behaviors within a student's control — including attending class, taking notes, reading the textbook, and studying the material on a regular basis. I've known many demotivated students who felt their daily efforts were overshadowed by the emphasis on exams.

Developing a comprehensive evaluation process

In April and August of 1995, I had the pleasure of working with a panel of evaluation experts to develop a set of measurement guidelines for the National Safety Council and the Centers for Disease Control. Our mission was to develop a handbook of practical guidelines that field personnel can use to evaluate the impact of an intervention to improve safety on family and commercial farms.

We agreed that evaluation was essential to hold people accountable for achieving program objectives. This pertains particularly to those developing and implementing the intervention. The evaluation process should measure whether intervention procedures: (a) are consistent with relevant principles and mission statements of the organization; (b) reach the desired audience and are implemented as planned; and (c) are efficient and effective. In sum, a complete evaluation process should assess how an intervention was conceived, designed, and implemented, and how efficient and effective it was.

Figure 18.1 summarizes our panel's deliberations on how to evaluate intervention impact. It integrates the primary issues discussed so far in this chapter. Lower levels of the hierarchy represent process activities needed to improve the higher-level outcomes of a safer environment and ultimate injury reduction. Immediate causes of injury reduction are changes in environment or behavior — or both.

Let's pause for a moment to consider the cause-and-effect connection between process and outcome. Behavior can be viewed as an outcome, shaped by a process that pursues changes in employee knowledge, perceptions, or attitudes. In this case, the behavior-change goal depends on employee participation in an intervention aimed at influencing a person state. Of course, intervention processes can be designed to circumvent person states and directly change behavior to reduce injuries, as discussed in Part 3 of this text.

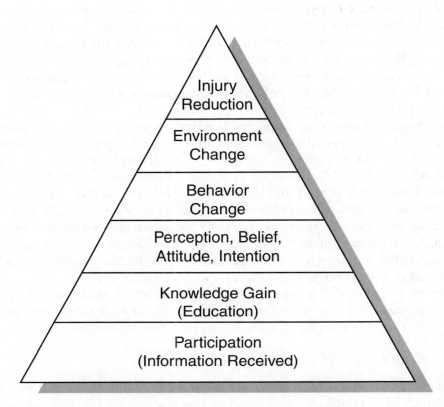

Figure 18.1 Measures of intervention impact vary according to remoteness from immediate injury causation.

Figure 18.1 points out the relativity of process and outcome. An education process, for example, can lead to behavior change (an outcome), while a process to change behaviors might result in outcome changes to the environment, say improved housekeeping. Completing a work process in a safer environment can effect the ultimate outcome — fewer injuries.

Figure 18.1 also reflects the three basic areas requiring attention for injury prevention — environment, behavior, and person. This is, of course, the Safety Triad introduced in Chapter 2 to categorize intervention strategies and referred to later in Chapter 14 to classify different types of actively caring behaviors. The hierarchical levels of intervention impact in Figure 18.1 reflect one or more of these three domains and suggest a particular approach to measurement. Changes in environments and behaviors can be assessed directly through systematic observation, but changes in knowledge, perceptions, beliefs, attitudes, and intentions are only accessible indirectly through survey techniques, usually questionnaires. Let's review these three basic areas of evaluation.

What to measure?

Most safety interventions focus on either environmental conditions — including engineering controls — or human conditions, as reflected in employees' perceptions, attitudes, or behaviors. It might seem reasonable to evaluate change only in the area we have targeted — environment, behavior, or person state. When the target is corporate culture, employee perceptions or attitudes are typically evaluated. If behavior change is the focus, then behaviors are observed and analyzed in terms of their frequency, rate, duration, or percentage of occurrence as reviewed in Chapter 8. When environments or engineering technologies are evaluated, mechanical, electrical, chemical, or structural measurements are taken.

I have heard culture-change consultants advocate perception surveys in place of environmental audits. Presentations on behavior-based safety emphasize direct observations of work practices, often in lieu of the subjective evaluation of personal perceptions and attitudes. Given the need, however, for employees to "feel good" about a behavior-based safety process and their need to participate continuously in managing and monitoring this process, I think it's obvious we need to check perceptions and attitudes *and* ongoing behaviors. For example, a comprehensive evaluation of a simple change in equipment design should probably include an assessment of relevant human factors like employees' work behaviors around the new equipment and their attitudes and perceptions regarding the equipment change.

I hope you can see that a comprehensive evaluation for safety requires a three-way audit process covering environmental conditions, safety-related behaviors, and person states such as perceptions, attitudes, beliefs, and intentions.

Evaluating environmental conditions

In many ways, environmental audits are the easiest and most acceptable type of evaluation. In fact, regular environmental or housekeeping audits are already standard practice at most companies. These evaluations can often be improved by involving more employees in designing audit forms, conducting systematic and regular assessments, and posting the results in relevant work areas.

Figure 18.2 depicts a generic environmental checklist for safety that can be used to graph for public display the percentage of safe conditions and the percentage of potential corrective actions taken for at-risk tools, equipment, or operating conditions. My associates at Safety Performance Solutions typically teach work teams the rationale behind the environmental checklist and then assist them in applying the checklist in their plant. Employees then customize the checklist and graphing procedures for their particular work areas. Regular audits and feedback sessions increase accountability for environmental factors that can be changed to prevent an injury.

The property damage incident. A provocative book by Bird and Germain (1997) focuses on environmental assessment, in particular, the need to investigate thoroughly the "property damage accident." Then the property damage needs to be fixed in order to prevent workplace injury. The authors claim the investigation and correction of property damage or property in need of repair are key to improving workplace safety. Yet, the property damage incident is sorely overlooked.

If you're underwhelmed by this so called "missing link," I understand. I felt the same when Frank Bird first related his passionate thoughts about the property damage accident. I did not understand the profound implications of this concept until reading his book and discussing it with line workers. For example, when I introduce the property damage incident at my workshops and seminars, line workers in attendance

| Observer:_____Date:_____ Time: _____ |
| Department: _____ Building: _____ Floor: _____ Area: _____ |

Operating Conditions/Tools & Equip.	Safe	At-Risk	*Corrective Actions Taken
Electrical wiring (properly enclosed)			
Air nozzles (limited to 30 P.S.I.)			
Chemicals (exposure concern)			
Eyewash station			
Emergency shower			
Barricades (in place where necessary)			
Storage of materials (neat/safe)			
Hazard Communication labels (appropriate)			
Floors (dry)			
Exits, aisles, sidewalks and walkways (clear of debris)			
Lighting (adequate)			
Housekeeping (satisfactory)			
Tools (safe operating condition)			
Guards (adequate and in place)			
Fire extinguisher (monthly inspection)			
Fire extinguisher (in appropriate location)			
GoJo (safe operation)			
GoJo driver (license in possession)			
Tow truck (safe operation)			
Tow truck driver (license in possession)			
Chairs in (safe condition)			
Totals			

Percent Safe Conditions: $\dfrac{\text{Total Safe Observations}}{\text{Total Safe Observations + At-Risk Observations}}$ x 100=_____%

Percent Corrective Actions Taken: $\dfrac{\text{Total Corrective Actions Taken:}}{\text{Total At-Risk Observations}}$ x 100=_____%

* Please list and define the corrective actions taken on back of this sheet.

Figure 18.2 An environmental checklist can be used to evaluate the safety of tools, equipment, and operating conditions.

show special interest. They often testify to the extreme amount of property damage at their work sites, including stockpiles of broken ladders, tools in disrepair, machine guards that don't work properly, and dents in equipment, walls, and vehicles. Each dent signals an incident, perhaps a near hit, that was not analyzed.

Front-line workers also verify the dramatic impact of property damage on their work demeanor which, in turn, influences their attitude about safety. To them, unrepaired property damage signifies that "Management doesn't care about our work situation," or "It's okay to damage property as long as we meet production demands."

An industrial example. Let me tell you a true story to illustrate how a focus on property damage can make a difference. Walking along a scaffold, a worker slipped on a metal plate and almost fell several stories to his death. Fortunately, he was able to catch himself with his arms and pull himself back onto the walkway. Members of the safety committee decided to do more than the typical "reactive investigation" of this incident. They did not simply blame the welder responsible for securing the plate. Instead, they looked for other contributing factors to prevent similar mishaps.

Guess what they discovered? At least a dozen people had slipped on that same loose plate and said nothing about it. No one reported a near hit. They did not want to report a "near miss," implying careless or thoughtless behavior. However, if the loose plate had been reported as property damage that needed immediate repair, the idea of individual blame would have been removed. Thus, not to report such property damage and thus assure correction should be considered careless and thoughtless.

Removing personal blame from incidents that set the stage for personal injury will enable more proactive reporting, evaluating, and correcting. When your periodic environmental audits show less and less property damage, you can be assured you are preventing injuries. In fact, I'm convinced this is actually a more reliable and valid metric for safety improvement than the standard injury and illness rates derived from employees' self reports and visits to the plant infirmary. So a comprehensive safety measurement system should include systematic audits of damage to the work environment. The repair of environmental damage should be continuously tracked as an ongoing measure of safety improvement.

Evaluating work practices

The systematic auditing of work practices was the theme of Chapters 8, 9, and 12. In Chapter 8, I introduced the overall DO IT process — "D" for define target behaviors, "O" for observe target behaviors, "I" for intervene to increase safe behavior or decrease at-risk behavior, and "T" for test (or evaluate) the impact of your intervention. How to develop two types of observation checklists was discussed in Chapter 8 — a generic version for basic work practices applicable anywhere, such as prescribed lifting techniques and the use of certain personal protective equipment (see Figures 8.12 and 8.13), and a job-specific checklist for particular tasks, like the safe driving checklist my daughter and I developed.

The coaching process detailed in Chapter 12 also discussed how to develop and apply both generic and job-specific checklists for one-on-one observation and feedback sessions with coworkers. As mentioned previously, using a behavioral checklist to observe and evaluate ongoing work practices is the type of performance appraisal that can lead to continuous improvement.

Chapter 9 on "Behavioral Safety Analysis" was all about evaluation from the perspective of work practices. A series of ten questions was proposed for conducting a step-by-step examination of the situational, social, and personal factors influencing at-risk behavior. Answers to these questions (see Figure 9.4) provide direction for deriving the most cost-effective corrective action plan.

Evaluating person factors

As discussed earlier in this text, person factors refer to subjective or internal aspects of people. They are reflected in commonly used terms like attitude, perception, feeling, intention, value, intelligence, cognitive style, and personality trait. You can find many surveys that measure specific person factors of target populations ranging from children to adults. Some of these factors are presumed to be *traits*, others are considered *states.* It is important to understand the difference when you consider the evaluation potential of a particular survey.

Person traits. Theoretically, traits are relatively permanent characteristics of people; they don't vary much over time or across situations. Because traits are relatively permanent, questionnaires that measure them cannot gauge the impact or progress of a culture-change intervention. Trait measures serve as a tool to teach individual differences but, in safety management, their application is limited to selecting people for certain job assignments. This is very risky, though, and not very effective, as discussed in Chapter 1.

Person states. Person states are characteristics that can change from moment to moment, depending on situations and personal interactions (as discussed in Chapter 15). When our goals are thwarted, for example, we can be in a state of frustration. When experiences lead us to believe we have little control over events around us, we can be in a state of apathy or helplessness. Person states can influence behaviors. Frustration, for example, often provokes aggressive behavior, and perceptions of helplessness inhibit constructive behavior or facilitate inactivity.

In contrast, certain life experiences can affect positive person states, such as optimism, personal control, self-confidence, and belonging. These, in turn, boost constructive behavior. This was the indirect approach to increasing actively caring behavior discussed in Chapter 16. The woman in Figure 18.3 is in a positive person state referred to as optimism. She might drive her friends crazy, but research has shown that healthier and happier people are more often in this state. Plus, as I discussed earlier in Chapter 15, optimistic people are more likely to actively care for the health or safety of others.

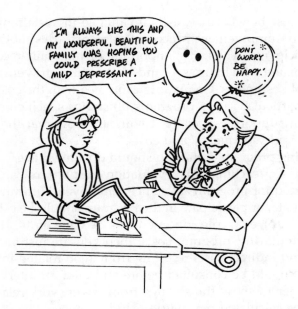

Figure 18.3 An optimistic person state facilitates happiness, perseverance, achievement, health, and actively caring.

Measures of person states can be used to evaluate perceptions of culture change and to pinpoint areas of a culture that need special intervention attention. Like most culture surveys, our Safety Culture Survey asks participants to answer questions on a five-point continuum (from highly disagree to highly agree) about their perceptions of the safety culture. Issues include the perceived amount of management support for safety, the willingness of employees to correct at-risk situations and look out for the safety of coworkers, the perceived risk level of the participant's job, and the nature of interpersonal consequences following an injury.

Our survey also measures factors that increase one's willingness to actively care for another person's safety. These include self-esteem, belonging, and empowerment as detailed in Chapter 15. Sample items from our survey that measure the actively caring person states are given in Chapter 15. They were adapted from professional measures of these characteristics.

Figure 18.4 contains 20 items from the safety perception and attitude portion of our survey. You'll note nothing very special about the items in this scale. They ask employees to react to straightforward statements about safety management and improvement.

You could compare employees' reactions to the items in Figure 18.4 before and after implementing a safety improvement process. Studying reactions prior to an intervention helps identify issues or work areas needing special attention. This information can lead you to choose a particular intervention approach or to customize one. Data from a baseline perception survey might even indicate that a culture is not ready for a given intervention process, suggesting the need for more education and discussion to get employees to "buy in."

Evaluating costs and benefits

A comprehensive cost–benefit analysis is invaluable in sustaining top-management support for a safety-improvement process. It also provides motivating feedback to the program participants. Thus, it's important to maintain records of direct and indirect costs associated with injuries — and with injury prevention — even if these calculations are only estimates. Comparing estimates with the costs of implementing and maintaining particular safety programs illustrates specific benefits and justifies continued program support, especially if you can show that the program has substantially reduced injury frequency and costs.

When calculating program costs, you should document every expense, including promotional materials, teaching aids, evaluation supplies, rewards, media expenditures, and wages paid for program assistance. Employees' time away from the job to plan, present, evaluate, or participate in the program should be estimated, even if the time is voluntary — for example, on evenings or weekends. If you are comprehensive when calculating program costs, then you are justified in estimating the numerous direct and indirect costs resulting from a job-related injury.

Injury records should be consulted before and after an intervention process has been started in order to show the savings from fewer work-related injuries. Direct costs that should be calculated per injury include:

- Wages paid to absent employees (workers' compensation)
- Property damage

	Highly Disagree	Disagree	Not Sure	Agree	Highly Agree
1. The risk level of my job concerns me quite a bit.	1	2	3	4	5
2. When told about safety hazards, supervisors are appreciative and try to correct them quickly.	1	2	3	4	5
3. My immediate supervisor is well informed about relevant safety issues.	1	2	3	4	5
4. It is the responsibility of each employee to seek out opportunities to prevent injury.	1	2	3	4	5
5. At my plant, work productivity and quality usually have a higher priority than work safety.	1	2	3	4	5
6. The managers in my plant really care about safety and try to reduce risk levels as much as possible.	1	2	3	4	5
7. When I see a potential safety hazard (e.g., oil spill), I am willing to correct it myself if possible.	1	2	3	4	5
8. Management places most of the blame for an accident on the injured employee.	1	2	3	4	5
9. "Near misses" are consistently reported and investigated at our plant.	1	2	3	4	5
10. I am willing to warn my coworkers about working unsafely.	1	2	3	4	5
11. Employees seen behaving unsafely in my department are usually given corrective feedback by their coworkers.	1	2	3	4	5
12. Compared to other plants, I think mine is rather risky.	1	2	3	4	5
13. Working safely is the number one priority in my plant.	1	2	3	4	5
14. I have received adequate job safety training.	1	2	3	4	5
15. Many first aid cases in my plant go unreported.	1	2	3	4	5
16. Information needed to work safely is made available to all employees.	1	2	3	4	5
17. Management here seems genuinely interested in reducing injury rates.	1	2	3	4	5
18. Safety audits are conducted regularly in my department to check the use of personal protective equipment.	1	2	3	4	5
19. I know how to do my job safely.	1	2	3	4	5
20. Most employees in my group would not feel comfortable if their work practices were observed and recorded by a coworker.	1	2	3	4	5

Figure 18.4 These questionnaire items measure personal perception regarding the safety of an organization and were selected from the Safety Culture Survey developed by Safety Performance Solutions, Inc. With permission.

- Medical expenses
- Physical and vocational rehabilitation costs
- Survivor benefits

These direct costs may be the proverbial tip of the iceberg when considering the indirect or hidden costs of business disruptions caused by a loss-time injury. However, indirect costs can be difficult or impossible to calculate. You should, however, try to estimate such costs in these categories:

- Overtime pay used to cover the work of an injured employee
- Scheduling work tasks to cover for an injured employee
- Additional administrative hassles, extra wages, training time, and inefficient work associated with temporary replacements
- Special costs of losing a skilled employee
- Extra time from work supervisors to schedule shift changes, temporary replacements, or employee training necessitated by the absence of an injured worker
- Retraining and readjusting for employees returning to work after an extended absence (A permanent disability from the injury might call for a new job assignment.)
- Special costs for extensive recruitment procedures and on-the-job training for permanent replacements for injured employees who do not return to work or who return with a permanent disability
- Special administrative costs to investigate and document the incident and medical treatments for compliance with state workers' compensation laws and with other state and federal regulations, such as OSHA standards

Considering the direct and indirect costs to a company from work-related injury is overwhelming in at least two respects. It's certainly an intimidating chore to estimate these costs, and it's stunning to think that the corporate losses from one employee's injury can be so great. These dollars clearly justify considerable intervention activity. Just anticipating the negative consequences from a work-related injury should motivate support and participation in proactive efforts. This is the first critical step in "selling" safety — the theme of the next chapter.

You can't measure everything

Deming (1991, 1992) condemned grades and performance appraisals because they provide a limited picture of an individual's contributions and potential. They might also constrain the number and type of interventions used to improve the quality of a work culture. If, for example, the only procedures implemented to improve safety are those that allow for objective measurement, the number and quality of safety interventions are severely restricted.

In Chapter 16, for example, I discussed a number of ways to increase actively caring behaviors directly, through applications of learning and social influence principles, and indirectly, through improving the five person states that increase willingness to actively care. It's impractical and impossible to measure the impact of many of these interventions. Should we avoid doing so just because we cannot measure their occurrence and impact?

Dr. Deming explained there are many things we should do for continuous improvement without attempting to measure their impact. We should not do these things only to influence performance indicators, but because they are the right things to do for people. You might never be able to measure the impact of treating an employee with special respect and dignity, but you do it anyway. Such treatment may, in fact, contribute to achieving a Total Safety Culture but you'll never know it. Likewise, you'll never know how many injuries you prevent with proactive actively caring

behaviors, and you'll never know how much actively caring behavior you will promote by taking even small steps to increase coworkers' self-esteem, empowerment,
and sense of belonging. You need to continue doing these things anyway. Many things
that cannot be measured and rewarded still need to get done.

In conclusion

At the start of this book, I explained the fallacy of basing decisions on common sense.
Rather than adopt intervention programs that sound good, we need to use procedures
that work. But how do we know what works? Of course, you know the answer to
this question. Only through rigorous program evaluation can we know whether an
intervention is worth pursuing. Now comes the more difficult question. What kind
of program evaluation is most appropriate for a particular situation?

Actually, every chapter of this text has addressed program evaluation in one way
or another. Early on, I explained the need for achievement-oriented methods to keep
score of your safety efforts. This enables people to consider safety in the same work-
to-achieve context as production and quality. This implies, of course, the need for
program evaluation numbers people can understand and learn from. This is how
evaluation leads to continuous improvement.

The information presented in this text is founded on rigorous evaluation, not
common sense. Evaluation techniques used in published research are, indeed, more
rigorous and complex in terms of reliability, validity, and statistical analysis than those
needed for continuous improvement of real-world safety programs. The basic principles and issues presented in this chapter, however, are relevant to both researchers
(seeking to contribute to professional scholarship) and practitioners (seeking continuous improvement of an intervention process).

To publish their findings, researchers need to demonstrate reliability and validity
of their measures and find statistical significance. However, they can and do ignore
several evaluation principles presented in this chapter. For example, their measures
typically target only one dimension (environment, behavior, or person factors), are
short-term (applied for a limited number of observation sessions), are subjected to
statistical transformations and analyses that take substantial time to complete and are
not readily understood by the average person, and often do not include a cost–benefit
analysis. You see, reports of their procedures and results only need to be understood
and appreciated by a select, often esoteric, group of professionals who specialize in
the particular issue or problem addressed by the research.

However, you cannot overlook the basic principles presented in this chapter when
evaluating practical interventions to achieve continuous improvement. Data collection
procedures and statistical analyses often can be less rigorous, but safety practitioners
need to address several important issues often bypassed by professional researchers.
Specifically, they need to

1. Define the level of performance targeted by the intervention, while appreciat-
    ing limitations in attacking individual vs. organizational performance.
2. Use measures for the three dimensions of safety improvement — environ-
    ment, behavior, and person factors.

3. Apply process measures periodically over the long term, especially checks on environmental conditions and work practices.
4. Include a cost–benefit analysis to justify continued intervention and evaluation efforts.
5. Keep score with numbers that are both meaningful to all program participants and provide direction for intervention refinement.

These last two principles are critical to meeting the challenge addressed in the next chapter — obtaining and maintaining support for an effective intervention process.

chapter nineteen

Obtaining and maintaining involvement

You cannot effectively put to use the principles in this book without ongoing support from both managers and employees. This chapter focuses on ways to initiate and maintain that support, including ways to promote leadership, build commitment and involvement, expand the scope of interventions, reduce active resistance, and sustain momentum.

"Character consists of what you do on the third and fourth tries." — James Michener

Culture change is never quick, never easy. The "quick-fix" illustrated in Figure 19.1 is clearly ridiculous. As absurd as this notion is, it comes to us naturally. We want speedy solutions to difficult challenges. It's easy to lose patience, enthusiasm, and optimism along the way. After all, our society demands immediate gratification —

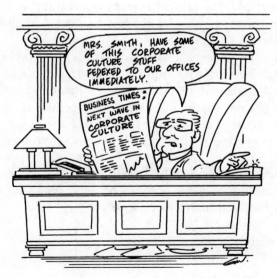

Fig 19.1 There is no quick-fix solution to culture change.

just look at all the movies and television shows that begin with dramatic problems and come to happy endings within 30 to 90 minutes. Plus, the faster we solve any problem, the sooner we experience rewarding positive consequences.

This chapter brings us to the point of pulling things together. I discuss the broad challenge of initiating a culture-change process aimed at achieving a Total Safety Culture. First, come general guidelines for starting a process and maintaining support. Then, I address concepts of leadership, communication, and resistance. You will not find step-by-step cookbook procedures here; a generic recipe is just not available. Instead, take the principles and procedures presented in prior chapters, add the information found here, and you'll be well on your way to an innovative experience in safety improvement.

Starting the process

Management support

You cannot do without it. How many times have you heard "Whatever management really pushes and supports will happen"? Implicitly, "Whatever upper management does not push and does not support will fail." If managers emphasize housekeeping, quality control, or cost-reduction, improvements in these areas are likely to follow. Strong top-down support, involvement, and commitment alone will not make a campaign succeed, but they are essential ingredients. Plus, management and labor must collaborate to make the process work.

Creating a safety steering team

A Safety Steering Team plays a critical role in developing a Total Safety Culture, providing policy-making, oversight, and general support. All this is simply more than any one person can handle.

Before creating a Safety Steering Team, however, it's important to look at the existing committee structure in your organization. You don't want to duplicate the efforts of the safety department or some other relevant standing committee. For example, a current employee team might be able to take on the responsibility of coordinating efforts to achieve a Total Safety Culture.

Careful planning is needed to determine the answers to these questions:

- What is the mission of the Safety Steering Team?
- What are the ground rules for how it operates? (See Chapter 17.)
- What are the group's limitations or restrictions?
- What are the priorities?
- Who should be on this team?

Developing evaluation procedures

"Did it do any good?" This is the central question the Safety Steering Team must be prepared to answer about any intervention. Chapter 18 offered guidelines for evaluating impact. At the start of an evaluation process, these questions need to be answered:

- What indicators should we look at — behaviors, attitudes, opinions, or outcomes?
- When should we measure?
- What types of data should we collect and analyze?
- What is the cost of this evaluation process?
- How should we summarize and display results?

Setting up an education and training process

Ensuring that employees learn key principles and procedures to improve safety is a major responsibility for the Safety Steering Team. At the minimum, the following elements should be incorporated into planning an effective education and training program:

- Develop education content and procedures.
- Plan the education and training process.
- Plan for follow-up sessions.
- Identify and prepare instructors.
- Measure the impact of the program.

Let's discuss each of these elements in a bit more detail, keeping in mind that my suggestions need to be customized at the plant level to get the most "bang for your buck."

Identifying and preparing instructors. Selecting the right instructors is critical because teaching is at the heart of effective education and training. If the teachers do a poor job, they undermine other training tools such as videos and booklets. You should consider these factors when choosing instructors:

- Prior experience in educating or training
- Current level of teaching ability (aptitude and achievement)
- Credibility with employees to be educated
- Level of motivation and interest in doing the instruction
- Prior familiarity with psychology, especially behavior-based principles
- Belief that the principles and procedures can help achieve a Total Safety Culture

To help prepare for their task, selected teachers will need to understand the principles and relevant procedures in this text so they can represent them accurately to the participants; feel comfortable with the specific process of the plant-wide education and training which, ideally, they will help to develop; practice basic communication skills; demonstrate leadership at meetings; and learn how to facilitate discussions — particularly if they have little experience at stand-up training and small-group meetings.

In-house training staff can help volunteers build their teaching skills. These topics are often covered in various corporate training programs. Plus, instructional programs are readily available from outside vendors or consultants.*

* My associates at Safety Performance Solutions (SPS) provide education and training, and guide organizations through the entire process reviewed here. For more information write Safety Performance Solutions, 1007 N. Main St., Blacksburg, VA 24060, call (540) 951-SAFE (7233), e-mail safety@safetyperformance.com, or visit our website at www.safetyperformance.com.

Developing course content. When considering the specific topics to include in each instructional session, you need to address these points:

- What are the specific goals of a particular session — for example, to teach principles, train procedures, or build commitment and motivation?
- In addition to this text, what sources are available for relevant content and support, such as local case studies of behavior-based safety?
- What relevant films, videotapes, and other instructional materials are available?*
- To meet session goals, what key content points should be covered, and in what order?
- What specific plant facts, statistics, and case studies can be incorporated into the session?
- How much information can be covered effectively in one session?

Involve your selected instructors as much as possible in developing the specific education and training plan.

Planning the instructional process. "Everything was covered but nobody paid much attention." This is a common complaint about education or training. The translation is that good content is important, but not sufficient. You've got to "package" your content and present it in a way that hits home with participants. Obviously, you want them to practice what is preached. Most instructors know their material; the challenge lies in conveying that knowledge. How do you get your message across? Here are some points to consider (for additional practical information on effective group presentation, see Drebinger, 2000):

- An interactive/participative approach is typically more effective than a "top-down" lecture coming from the podium.
- Like a good pitcher, change speeds. Do not rely on one pitch, one way of presenting information.
- It's easier to involve small groups of participants than large ones.
- Regardless of the main objective of a session, some initial awareness raising makes participants more receptive to the content.
- Integrate demonstrations into the program.
- If possible, have participants practice the skill taught with appropriate feedback in the classroom or on the job.
- Resolve those administrative questions, including where and when the instructional sessions should be held, and how long they should take.

Evaluating effectiveness. As covered in Chapter 18, you cannot overlook measurement. At this point in the overall intervention process, you need to determine impact of education and training on participants' knowledge, skill, and attitudes.

Knowledge of content can be assessed the old-fashioned way, through written tests given at the end of a session. Skills can be evaluated by systematic behavioral

---

* A variety of instructional materials on behavior-based safety and actively caring, including videotapes, audiotapes, and facilitator guides are available through Safety Performance Solutions, Inc.

observation in the classroom or out in the workplace. Participants' reactions to the session can be measured with brief questionnaires. For this you should keep in mind

- Brevity
- Choice and complexity of wording
- Combining objective ratings and written comments

Sustaining the process

Continued upper-management support. Many safety programs get a big send-off, only to drop off the radar screen. Then, it's "out of sight, out of mind" as some new program is pushed. This is why safety is often derided for its "flavor of the month" approach. So how do we sustain a safety process? (Note that I prefer the concept of "process" to "program" here because processes flow on while programs begin and end.) First and foremost, we need continued and visible support from top management. If management endorses the process on an ongoing basis, it can become integrated into normal plant operations.

The Safety Steering Team needs to work hard to convince managers that their commitment is fundamental to the process — not only to get it going, but also to keep it going. Here are some thoughts on maintaining that all-important backing of top managers:

- First, you need to gain access to upper management. Identify a manager to champion your cause in the executive offices. Bring him or her into the loop; ask him or her to attend all team meetings.
- Keep managers informed. Submit team reports to them on a regular basis but do not overwhelm busy managers with minutiae.
- Keep managers involved. Solicit their comments and "concerns" about the process you have underway. Of course, you should be doing this with all levels of the organization to create a top-to-bottom sense of ownership.
- Promote and market your efforts. Publish articles and announcements about the safety process in the employee newsletter on a regular basis.
- Keep at it. Identify the benefits of your process and continue to "sell" them to upper management.

Follow-up instruction/booster sessions

Even with ongoing support, a comprehensive safety improvement process cannot succeed without carefully planned follow-up instruction. From time to time, education and training content must be updated to reflect changes in plant conditions, the use of new machines or protective equipment, and the like. Do not delay in keeping pace with change; what is being taught should correspond exactly to current plant conditions. Follow-up education and training involve these issues:

- When and how should basic instruction be repeated for new employees?*
- What are the objectives of follow-up instruction?

---

* For information on an interactive computer instructional program with on-line access, contact Safety Performance Solutions, Inc., 1007 N. Main St., Blacksburg, VA 24060. Call (540) 951-7233, or e-mail safety@ safetyperformance.com

- How should new material be integrated?
- How often should follow-up sessions occur?
- What should be the content?
- How should the material be presented — film, lecture, on-the-job training, discussion groups, audio tapes, interactive computer program?
- How can monthly safety talks in team meetings be used as boosters or activators?

Troubleshooting and fine-tuning

Once a safety achievement process is up and running, the Safety Steering Team confronts the responsibility of fine-tuning the procedures. This is based on ongoing evaluations. If the process is going to be sustained, employees and managers must perceive it as current — "state of the art" — in terms of content, adaptability, and responsiveness. It simply cannot be "frozen" nor left unattended. You cannot "wind up" a process at the start and expect it to run forever like that battery-powered bunny. Some keys to fine-tuning include:

- Discuss the impact — is it working? What do the data from participants' reaction sheets, as well as other measures, tell us?
- Identify strengths and weaknesses. Based on the data, which elements should be kept, changed (and how), or replaced?
- Cope with change. Be sure all those affected by the process are fully informed about changes when they occur. Ideally, all participants should be actively involved in trouble-shooting and fine-tuning interventions.

Cultivating continuous support

Starting a safety improvement process and maintaining it over the long term requires the three essential support processes depicted in Figure 19.2. Communication and recognition are covered in Chapter 13. Here I want to focus on leadership. Leaders are needed to champion new principles and procedures. In fact, leadership makes the difference between a "flavor of the month" safety initiative and a long-term continuous improvement process.

My colleagues and I at Safety Performance Solutions have seen the principles and procedures presented in this book lead to remarkable success and, eventually, a Total Safety Culture. All too often, however, we have seen good intentions and superb introductory instruction fizzle out and go nowhere. Why? It's a matter of leadership. You can launch a process with excellent education and training, but you cannot keep the momentum going without individuals who provide energy, enthusiasm, and the right example. This section covers some essentials of effective leadership.

Where are the safety leaders?

First, we have to find the leaders. Who are they? The traditional definition of one person exerting influence over a group does not quite work for safety. Ask any safety manager who has been expected to do it all. To achieve a Total Safety Culture, everyone needs to accept a leadership role in reducing injuries. Everyone needs to feel responsible for safety and go beyond the call of duty to protect others. This

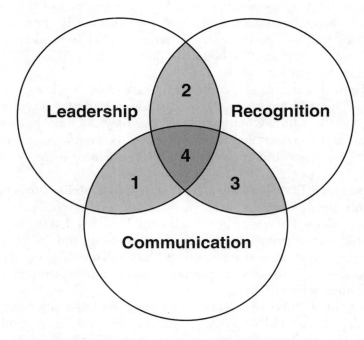

1. Leaders *communicate* effectively.
2. Leaders *recognize* desired performance.
3. *Recognition* is *communicated* effectively.
4. Leaders *recognize* desired performance
   effectively through a variety of
   communication channels.

Figure 19.2 Continuous improvement depends on three support systems.

requires leadership skills, including giving supportive feedback for another person's safe behavior and constructive feedback for at-risk behavior.

Psychologists have studied leadership rigorously for over 50 years in an attempt to define the traits and styles of good leaders. Still, many questions remain unanswered, making leadership more an art than a science. Several decades of research, however, have turned up some important answers, which we will now apply to safety.

Passion. The most successful leaders show energy, desire, passion, enthusiasm, and constant ambition to achieve. Passion to achieve a Total Safety Culture can be fueled by clarifying goals and tracking progress. Put a positive spin on safety, make it something to be achieved — not losses to avoid. Then, employees will be motivated to achieve shared safety goals just like they work toward production and quality goals. Making progress leads to the genuine belief that the process works. This fires up employees to continue the process.

Honesty and integrity. Effective leaders are open and trustworthy. A Total Safety Culture depends on open interpersonal conversation. This obviously requires honesty, integrity, and trust. It is useful for work groups to discuss ways to nurture these qualities in their culture. Take a look at certain environmental conditions, policies, and behaviors. Some arouse suspicions of hidden agendas, politics, and selfish aims. You can work to eliminate some of these trust-busters by first identifying them, discussing their purpose, and devising alternatives. While frankness is important in increasing trust, it's important to be tactful (*not* shown in Figure 19.3) when communicating an honest opinion.

Motivation. Because most people really care about reducing personal injuries, even to people they do not know, the motivation to lead others will spread naturally throughout a work culture when people believe they can have personal control over injuries. This occurs when they learn effective techniques to prevent injuries (as presented in Parts 3 and 4 of this text) and feel empowered to apply them (as covered in Part 5).

Self-confidence. Effective leaders trust in their own abilities to achieve. Education helps convince people they can achieve, but they need ongoing support and recognition for their efforts. For example, the self-confidence needed to give safety feedback can be initiated with appropriate education and training, and can be maintained with coaching, communication, and recognition. Notice that enhancing the three empowerment factors — self-efficacy, personal control, and optimism — discussed in Chapter 16 builds self-confidence.

Thinking skills. Successful leaders can integrate large amounts of information, interpret it objectively and coherently, and act decisively as a result. Constructive thinking skills evolve among team members when objective data are collected on the progress of safety interventions and used to refine or expand these processes and develop new ones.

When teams work through the DO IT process (as covered in Part 4), participants develop skills to evaluate behavioral data and use the information to make intervention

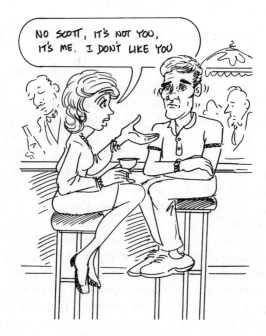

Figure 19.3 Candor should be delivered tactfully.

decisions. This is basic scientific thinking, the key to substituting profound knowledge for common sense. This mindful learning (Langer, 1997) and critical thinking lead to special expertise.

Expertise. To achieve a Total Safety Culture, everyone needs to understand the principles behind policies, rules, and interventions to improve safety. When employees teach these principles to coworkers, they develop the level of profound knowledge, expertise, and responsibility needed for exemplary leadership.

Flexibility. Successful leaders size up a situation, and adjust their style accordingly. At times, some groups and circumstances call for firm direction — an autocratic style. At other times, the same people might work better under a nondirective, hands-off approach — a democratic style. The best leaders are good at assessing people and situations, and then matching their behavior to fit the need.

Overcoming resistance to change

"How do we deal with people who resist change?"
"How do we get more people to participate?"

I frequently hear these questions at training seminars and workshops. First, let's face reality. Change is unpleasant for many people, and some are apt to react poorly. Change often threatens our "comfort zones" — those predictable daily routines we like to control. In fact, it takes a certain amount of personal security and leadership to try something new. A certain kind of risk taking is needed to lead change, and some people want no part of exploring the unknown.

We have all been in unfamiliar situations where we are not sure how to act. We feel awkward and uncomfortable. If someone gives us direction, helps increase our sense of control, it's easier to adjust. We might even help others deal with the change. Without leaders and adequate tools to cope with change, we might retreat, withdraw from the situation, or even actively resist the change.

So how do we deal with resistance? Simply put, we should teach people the skills and give them the tools to handle change, plus support those who set the right examples. This seems logical and intuitive, but it does not always happen. Instead, managers too often try to identify the malcontents and discipline them for not participating.

Let's try to better understand resistance by considering one of the classic awkward, strange situations thrust upon many of us — our first school dance. Remember it? For me, it was a high school homecoming dance in 1957.

Remember your first dance. Attending your first dance is like a rite of passage. If you were anything like me, you were a bit nervous about this change in your social world. You might have been prepared for it. Family, friends, and teachers probably told you what to expect. Maybe you even had dance lessons, but these "tools" did not make it any easier for some of us to participate.

Not for me, anyway. I did not participate, but I wanted to. Before the dance, I practiced how to ask a girl to dance. I took four, two-hour dance lessons at an Arthur Murray Dance Studio. I felt ready, but never once did I dance that night. I didn't feel too embarrassed, though, because there were so many others not dancing. As was the custom, boys stood on one side of the gym and the girls on the other.

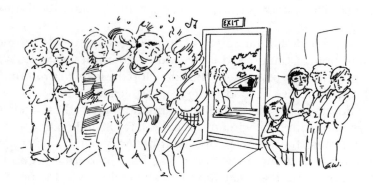

Figure 19.4 Different reactions to change can be seen at the high-school dance.

As illustrated in Figure 19.4, some kids were dancing and seemed to be having a great time. They danced almost every number and tried to lure others out on the floor. I could not be enticed, though. I hung back in my comfort zone but, at least, I was in the dance hall.

As illustrated in Figure 19.5, some students stood around in the parking lot, talking, drinking, and smoking cigarettes. These were the resisters. Some were *active* resisters. They stayed in their cars, never intending to enter the dance hall. Now and then, these guys started up their cars and cruised around town for awhile, then returned to the parking lot. They would persuade others to hop in their car, try some beer, smoke a cigarette, fool around, or cruise.

Levels of participation. There are essentially five ways of reacting to change — call them levels of participation — and they were all on display at the dance. First, there are the true leaders who get totally involved. They are the innovators — those who view change as necessary and an opportunity to improve. At the dance, they were the teenagers on the floor for almost every number. They had the most fun. They did not necessarily know what they were doing when it came to dancing, but they got out there and tried. They took a risk. They got totally involved and benefited most from the occasion. A dance might start with only a few of these "risk takers," but they often persuaded a number of others to get involved as the night wore on.

Some people want to change but need direction and support. They are motivated to participate but need models or leaders. At the dance, these were the kids who hung back at first. With a little encouragement, they danced a few numbers. By the end of the evening, you could not get them off the dance floor. They were now totally involved.

Most of us are at the third level of participation. We are ready to get involved, but we will stay in our comfort zones until we are directed *and* motivated to participate. It might look like we are resisting change, but not really. Call us neutral when it comes to our attitude about change. We just are not sure what to do. We need self-confidence that we can handle the change. We also need genuine support (positive recognition) when we try to participate. Once in a while, just getting started, or "breaking the ice," is enough to turn a passive observer into an active participant.

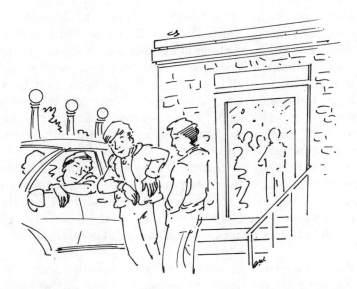

Figure 19.5 Some actively resist change while others follow.

For the most part, however, we stand on the sidelines and watch. This level of participation was represented by the boys and girls who lined each side of the gym.

Types of resistance. The final two levels of participation are passive and active resistance. Passive resisters perceive change as a problem. They complain a lot. They are critical and untrusting of something new imposed on them. They seem to see only the negative side of a new program, policy, or challenge. They rationalize their position by gathering with others at their same level of nonparticipation, and they grumble and whine about proposed changes or about others who are participating in a change effort. Their whining and complaining usually stops when participation in a new process is clearly enjoyed by the majority. Passive resisters are followers, and they will do what they see most people doing.

These are the teenagers who came to the dance because everyone else would be there, but they felt so insecure or anxious they did not enter the building. They looked for others hanging around outside and made fun of the silly dancing going on inside. Sometimes, these nonparticipants ran into an *active* resister.

Fortunately, active resisters are few in number, but it doesn't take many of these characters to slow down a change process. These individuals view change as a threat or an opportunity to resist. They see any change effort that was not their idea as a potential loss of personal control, and they often exert countercontrol to assert their control or freedom. Most parents observe this phenomenon when their children reach the "teens." Teenagers want to feel independent and, at times, will disobey their parents' directions — break the rules — to gain a sense of independence or self-control.

We all feel overly controlled at times and, perhaps, react to regain independence or assert personal freedom. Sometimes, our reactions are not thoughtful, caring, or safe. Active resisters feel the need to resist change, the status quo, or authority much of the time. This is partly because their contrary behavior brings them special attention — recognition for resisting.

Who gets the attention? Active resisters stand out and attract attention. Nonparticipants use them to rationalize their own commitment to comfort zones. Managers monitoring the workplace often hit them with discipline, but this can backfire. This makes the top-down control more obvious for resisters. Discipline builds their resentment of the system and makes it even less likely they will join the change process.

For some individuals, disciplinary attention only fuels their burning desire to exert independence and resist change. As a result, they might become more vigorous in recruiting others to oppose change. As I discussed in Chapter 11, top-down discipline (actually punishment) should be used sparingly if the ultimate purpose is total participation in an improvement process.

How were resistant teenagers brought inside to the dance? The harsh warnings of the school principal shouting from the steps did not work; neither did the one-on-one confrontation between one of the adult chaperones and the "leader of the pack." Whenever I saw a resister come inside, it was always the result of urging by another teenager. Peer pressure (or peer support) is still the most powerful motivator of human behavior.

Therefore, the best way to deal with resistance is usually to arrange for situations that enable or facilitate peer influence. Eventually, some of the resistant teenagers came into the building so they would not miss something. As depicted in Figure 19.6, they saw from their remote comfort zones that the people inside were really enjoying themselves, and they chose to participate.

The dance party will become more enticing as more and more teenagers dance. To increase such active involvement, the right kind of encouragement and support is needed. Will a motivational lecture from a teacher, counselor, concerned parent, or outside consultant make that happen? It might make a temporary difference but not over the long haul. The best way to deal with nonparticipation is usually to set up situations that allow for peer influence. This could mean managers do nothing more than support the change process and let peer pressure or support occur naturally.

In conclusion

This chapter began with a list of guidelines to initiate and sustain a culture-change process aimed at achieving a Total Safety Culture. Three support processes were identified to maintain employees' long-term commitment and involvement in a culture-change effort — leadership, communication, and recognition. Communication and recognition were discussed earlier in Chapter 13, so leadership received more attention here.

Psychologists find the best leaders are enthusiastic, honest, motivated, confident, analytical, informed, and flexible. Although it's common to see these characteristics described as permanent personality traits, it's certainly reasonable to assume they can be increased through education, communication, recognition, and involvement in a successful safety process. Thus, while it's useful to look for "natural" leaders when selecting members of a Safety Steering Team, it's important to realize that leadership qualities could be suppressed in some people by their lack of empowerment or sense of belonging. New safety processes and eventual culture change might bring out leaders you did not know existed in the work force.

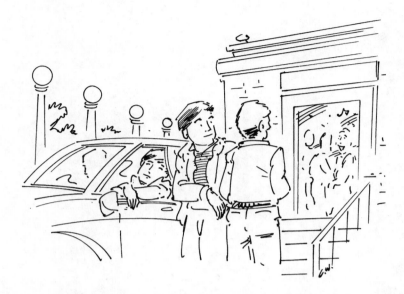

Figure 19.6 When a critical mass of the culture changes, others follow.

Involvement is key to so many aspects of building a Total Safety Culture and it can be increased many ways. Expect to see five levels of involvement:

1. Total involvement from innovators who see change as an opportunity to improve.
2. Individuals committed but not totally involved until direction and support are given.
3. People, usually the majority, ready but on the sidelines until prodded and encouraged by others.
4. Doubters who see change as a problem and use learned helplessness and cynicism as excuses to remain detached.
5. The active resisters who see change as an opportunity to resist, complain, and promote mistrust.

Active and passive resisters (categories 4 and 5) should be ignored, if possible. Recognize and support those willing to try the new process. Employees totally involved in the process (category 1) need to help individuals committed but not yet totally immersed (category 2). Then these two groups can work with the majority (category 3) who need examples to follow. You can see why it's important to cultivate leadership, communication, and recognition skills among the "true believers" in innovation. Turn these leaders loose and they will be your best recruiters to build the base of support for a Total Safety Culture.

chapter twenty

Reviewing the principles

This book summarizes principles for understanding the human dynamics of safety. When you use these principles to design, execute, evaluate, and continuously improve interventions to improve safety-related behaviors and attitudes, you are well on your way to achieving a Total Safety Culture.

"If you want to get a good idea, get a lot of ideas." — Linus Pauling

"How should we translate these concepts into real-world application?"
"Would you please put your theory into procedures or practices we could follow in our plant?"

I have heard questions like these at each of the Deming workshops I attended. They seemed to disappoint Dr. Deming (1991, 1992), who would assert that the purpose of the seminar was to teach theory and principles, not specific procedures. It was up to the participants to return to their own organizations and devise specific methods and procedures that fit their culture. Deming stressed the need to start with theory and then customize practices.

As Professor Deming well knew, and as I have discussed throughout this text, lasting improvement is built on specific procedures that fit the culture of an organization. Outside consultants can be invaluable, teaching appropriate principles and facilitating the implementation process, but if most of the employees do not understand and believe in the principles to begin with, well-intentioned efforts never take root.

The 50 principles

It all starts with theory. In this final chapter, I pull together 50 important principles that summarize the psychology of safety and lay the groundwork for building a Total Safety Culture. I know 50 sounds like a long list, but don't worry, I'll be brief. The principles will be familiar to you, having come from information already covered.

I hope you'll find the list useful as a review and as a starting point for developing your safety-enhancement process. Some of the principles focus on design and implementation. Others explain why we often fail in safety. Most can be used as guidelines for checking potential long-term benefits of a specific safety-improvement procedure. All will help you appreciate the complex human dynamics of safety and health promotion.

This is not a priority list. Do not read anything into the order of principles. What I hope is that you teach them to others. You *can* make a difference and bring about constructive culture change.

Principle 1: Safety should be internally — not externally — driven.

It's common to hear employees talk about safety in terms of OSHA — the Occupational Safety and Health Administration. It often seems they "do" safety more to satisfy the mandates of this outside regulatory agency than for themselves. This translates into perceptions of top-down control and performing to avoid penalties rather than to achieve success.

Ownership, commitment, and proactive behaviors are more likely when we work toward our own goals, not the government's. As discussed in Chapter 19, how we define programs and activities can influence attitudes that shape involvement. It makes sense to talk about corporate safety as a mission owned and achieved by the very people it benefits.

Principle 2: Culture change requires people to understand the principles and how to use them.

In Chapter 9, I distinguished between education and training and emphasized that long-term culture change requires both. Education focuses on theory or principles. Training gets into the specifics of how to turn principles into effective action. Role playing or one-on-one interaction is very important for training because participants get direct feedback on how they are executing procedures or processes.

Principle 3: Champions of a Total Safety Culture will emanate from those who teach the principles and procedures.

When people teach, they "walk the talk" and become champions of change. After more than 30 years of safety consulting, it's clear to me that success depends on the presence of these leaders. I have seen no better way to develop champions of a campaign than first to teach relevant theory and method, then show how others can be instructors, and finally allow opportunities for colleagues and coworkers to teach each other.

Principle 4: Leadership can be developed by teaching and demonstrating the characteristics of effective leaders.

Just because you believe in something does not guarantee you will be an effective champion of the cause. Leaders have certain characteristics, as discussed in Chapter 19, that can be taught to and cultivated in others. People need to understand the principles behind good leadership and the behaviors that reflect good leadership qualities. You can also learn by observing the leadership skills of others. When you see leaders in action, reward their exemplary behavior with quality recognition or rewarding feedback.

Principle 5: Focus recognition, education, and training on people reluctant but willing, rather than on those resisting.

As discussed in Chapter 19, people resist change for many reasons. Some feel insecure leaving their comfort zones. Some mistrust any change in policy or practice that was not their idea. Others balk for the special attention they get by resisting. It is usually a waste of time trying to force change on these folks. In fact, resistance hardens as more pressure is applied.

Principle 6: Giving people opportunities for choice can increase commitment, ownership, and involvement.

A basic reason for preferring the use of positive over negative consequences to motivate behavior (Chapter 11) is that people feel more free. They perceive more choice when working to achieve rewards than when working to avoid penalties. As illustrated in numerous laboratory experiments and field applications, increasing perceptions of choice lead to more motivation and involvement in the process (Chapter 16).

Principle 7: A Total Safety Culture requires continuous attention to factors in three domains: environment, behavior, and person.

Early on, I introduced the "Safety Triad" with behavior and person sides representing the psychology of safety. That is the focus of this book, but do not overlook the need for environmental change. The environment includes physical conditions and the general atmosphere or ambiance regarding safety. The behavioral safety analysis presented in Chapter 9 started with addressing ways to simplify the task through re-engineering. Thus, before addressing behavior change, it's critical to improve environmental conditions that can make a job more user friendly and ergonomically sound.

Principle 8: Do not count on common sense for safety improvement.

Most common sense is not common. It is biased by our subjective interpretation of unique experiences. As a researcher of psychological principles for more than 35 years, I have become quite committed to this basic principle (discussed in Chapter 2). Indeed, I have dedicated most of my career to discovering principles of human behavior through systematic application of the scientific method.

Principle 9: Safety incentive programs should focus on the process rather than outcomes.

One of the most frequent common-sense mistakes in safety management is the use of outcome-based incentive programs. Giving rewards for avoiding an injury seems reasonable and logical, but it readily leads to covering up minor injuries and a distorted picture of safety performance. The basic activator–behavior–consequence contingency (see Chapter 8 and Principle 18) demonstrates that safety incentives need

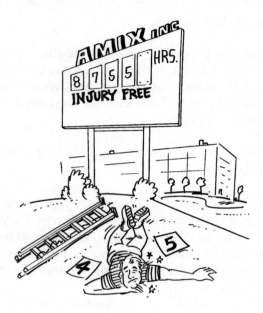

Figure 20.1 Focus on process to improve outcome statistics.

to focus on process activities, or safety-related behaviors. As illustrated in Figure 20.1, however, it's easy to get over-focused on outcome measures and overlook processes needed to achieve the outcome.

> *Principle 10: Safety should not be considered a priority but a value with no compromise.*

As discussed in Chapter 3, this is the ultimate vision. Safety becomes a value linked to every priority in the workplace or wherever we find ourselves. Priorities change according to circumstances; values are deep-seated personal beliefs beyond compromise.

> *Principle 11: Safety is a continuous fight with human nature.*

I know people who meet the behavioral criteria for holding safety as a value — they practice safety, teach it, go out of their way to actively care for the safety of others, but their numbers are few. Why? Because human nature (or natural motivating consequences, Chapter 11) typically encourages at-risk behavior.

We're talking about comfort, convenience, and expediency. When you compete with natural supportive consequences in order to teach, motivate, or change behavior, you're fighting human nature.

Principle 12: Behavior is learned from three basic processes: classical conditioning, operant conditioning, and observational learning.

Through naturally occurring consequences and planned instructional activities, we learn every day and we develop attitudes and emotional reactions to people, events, and environmental stimuli. The mechanisms for learning voluntary and involuntary behavior and emotions were reviewed in Chapter 8.

Principle 13: People view behavior as correct and appropriate to the degree they see others doing it.

Because personal experience often convinces us that "it's not going to happen to me," we need a powerful reason to perform safely when personal injury is improbable. So consider this: Everyone who sees you acting safely or at risk either learns a new behavior or thinks what you are doing is okay. Now, consider the vast number of people who observe your behavior every day. Our influence as a social model gives us special responsibility to go out of our way for safety.

Principle 14: People will blindly follow authority, even when the mandate runs counter to good judgment and social responsibility.

The fact that people often follow top-down rules without regard to potential risk is alarming. This puts special responsibility on managers and supervisors who give daily direction. These front-line leaders could signal, even subtly, the approval of at-risk behavior in order to reach production demands. People are apt to follow even implicit demands from their supervisor to whom they readily delegate responsibility for injury that could result from at-risk behavior.

Principle 15: Group participation can be enhanced by increasing personal responsibility, individual accountability, group cohesion, and interdependence.

Giving up personal responsibility for safety to another person (Principle 14) could be due to the lack of those factors needed for interdependent teamwork. Thus, workplace interventions and action plans need to be implemented with the aim of increasing an individual's perception of individual accountability and personal responsibility, including one's sense of group cohesion and interdependence (Chapter 17).

Principle 16: On-the-job observation and interpersonal feedback are key to achieving a Total Safety Culture.

Critical behavior checklists (Chapter 8) and communicating the results of checklist observations (Chapter 12) put this principle to work. Unlike the situation depicted in Figure 20.2, the observation and feedback process must be positive. Only then will this basic improvement tool spread throughout a work culture. The more people giving and receiving interpersonal feedback related to safety, the greater the improvement in safety-related behaviors and the more injuries prevented.

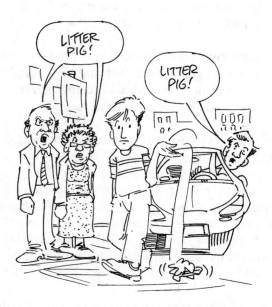

Figure 20.2 While some negative feedback seems warranted, it's unlikely
to have a beneficial effect.

*Principle 17: Behavior-based safety is a continuous DO IT process with D = Define
target behaviors, O = Observe target behaviors, I = Intervene to improve behaviors,
and T = Test impact of intervention.*

The four-step DO IT process enables continuous improvement through an objective behavior-focused approach. As detailed in Chapter 8, people need to decide on critical target behaviors to observe. After baseline observations are taken, an intervention is developed and implemented. By continuing to observe the target behaviors, the impact of the intervention program can be objectively evaluated. Results might suggest a need to refine the intervention, carry out another one, or define a different set of behaviors to work on. The next four principles provide guidance for designing behavior-change interventions.

Principle 18: Behavior is directed by activators and motivated by consequences.

External or internal events occurring before behavior (referred to as activators) only motivate to the extent they signal or specify consequences. Intentions and goals can motivate behavior if they stipulate positive or negative consequences. Understanding this principle is critical to developing effective behavior-change techniques.

Principle 19: Intervention impact is influenced by the amount of response information, participation, and social support, as well as external consequences.

Interventions that give specific instructions (response information) and get participants actively involved are likely to influence behavior and attitude change. If the intervention facilitates support from others, such as coworkers or family members, it can have lasting effects. Furthermore, people are more apt to develop internal motivation when external rewards or threats are relatively small and insufficient to completely justify the target behavior.

> *Principle 20: Extra and external consequences should not overjustify the target behavior.*

The various examples of positive consequences presented in Chapters 11 and 12 are not large nor expensive. For the reasons discussed previously, rewards should not provide complete justification for desired behavior. We don't want people complying with safety rules only to gain a reward or avoid a penalty. If that is the case, what happens when we take away the consequence, good or bad? We take away the reason to comply. This is why many people wear PPE at work, but rarely at home.

> *Principle 21: People are motivated to maximize positive consequences (rewards) and minimize negative consequences (costs).*

Of course, this principle relates to many behaviors. In Chapter 14, it was used to explain why people often do not rush to help in a crisis. If there are more perceived costs than benefits to intervening, actively caring behavior is unlikely. Therefore, a prime strategy for increasing safety and actively caring behaviors is to overcome the costs (negative consequences) with benefits (positive consequences). Various kinds of consequences are defined by the next principle.

> *Principle 22: Behavior is motivated by eight possible combinations of consequences: positive vs. negative, natural vs. extra, and internal vs. external.*

Understanding these characteristics (as explained in Chapter 11) can enable significant insights into the motivation behind observed behavior. Appreciating these various consequences can also suggest whether external intervention is called for to change behavior and what kind of intervention to implement.

Can you define the type of consequences motivating the biker in Figure 20.3? The odometer provides external and natural immediate feedback to the exerciser as he pedals. When he talks to himself while pedaling, he adds internal motivating feedback to the situation. His evaluation of the feedback determines whether the feedback is positive or negative.

> *Principle 23: Negative consequences have four undesirable side effects: escape, aggression, apathy, and countercontrol.*

How did you feel the last time you received a reprimand from a supervisor? Maybe, you felt like slinking away or taking a swipe at him. Chances are you did not go back to the job charged up. Perhaps, you wanted to do something to make him look bad. These and other undesirable side effects of using negative consequences are discussed in Chapter 11.

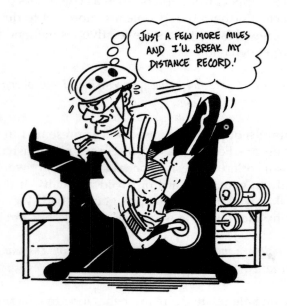

Figure 20.3 Natural immediate consequences can be very motivating.

Principle 24: Natural variation in behavior can lead to a belief that negative consequences have more impact than positive consequences.

Behavior fluctuates from good to bad for many reasons. Peak performance seldom can be sustained, and poor performance is almost bound to get better at some point. So if you praise someone and their performance falters, don't swear off positive feedback and don't overestimate the power of your reprimand if it seems to get some immediate results. The improvement was likely due to natural or "common cause" regression to the mean. Keep things in perspective. Remember, only with positive consequences can both behavior and attitude be improved.

Principle 25: Long-term behavior change requires people to change "inside" as well as "outside."

The psychology of safety requires us to consider both external behavior and internal person factors. Chapter 15 focused on the role of person states in influencing people to actively care for another person's safety and health. Chapter 16 showed how outside factors can be manipulated to influence these person states and, thus, increase actively caring behavior. A Total Safety Culture requires integrating both behavior-based and person-based psychology. The next several principles focus on understanding "inside" factors.

Principle 26: All perception is biased and reflects personal history, prejudices, motives, and expectations.

Appreciating this principle is key to understanding people and realizing the importance of actively listening to others before intervening. It also supports the need to depend on objective, systematic observation for knowledge rather than common sense (Principle 8).

It's important to realize the reciprocal relationship between perception and behavior. Perceptions influence actions and, in turn, actions influence perceptions. If we perceive risk, we will act to reduce it; by acting to reduce risk, we will become more aware of other risks.

Principle 27: Perceived risk is lowered when a hazard is perceived as familiar, understood, controllable, and preventable.

When people perceive a new risk, they adjust their behavior to avoid it. Call it "fear of the unknown." The reverse is also true. As discussed in Chapter 5, research has shown that hazards perceived as familiar, understood, controllable, and preventable are viewed as less risky. This is why many hazards are underestimated by employees.

Principle 28: The slogan "all injuries are preventable" is false and reduces perceived risk.

Frankly, I believe telling people all injuries are preventable insults their intelligence. They know better. It's difficult enough to anticipate and control all environmental and behavioral factors contributing to injuries, but controlling factors inside people is clearly impossible. The most critical problem with this popular slogan is that it can reduce the perception of risk. Hazards considered controllable and preventable are perceived as relatively risk free.

Principle 29: People compensate for increases in perceived safety by taking more risks.

As reviewed in Chapter 5, researchers have shown that some people will compensate for a decrease in perceived risk by performing more risky behavior. In other words, some people increase their tolerance for risk when feeling protected with a safety device. As shown in Figure 20.4, high technology safety engineering can give a false sense of security. This is not the case for people who hold safety as a value (Principle 10).

Principle 30: When people evaluate others they focus on internal factors; when evaluating personal performance, they focus on external factors.

As discussed in Chapter 6, this principle is termed "The Fundamental Attribution Error." It contributes to systematic bias whenever we attempt to evaluate others, from completing performance appraisals to conducting an injury investigation. Because we are quick to attribute internal (person-based) factors to other people's behavior, we tend to presume consistency in others because of permanent traits or personality characteristics. To explain injuries to other persons, we use expressions like "He's just careless," "She had the wrong attitude," and "They were not thinking like a team."

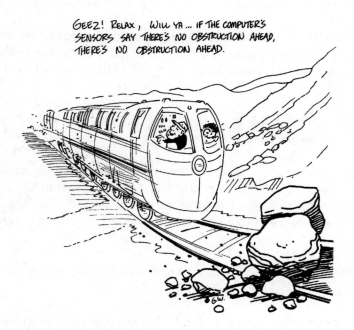

Figure 20.4 Technology can cause reduced perception of risk and increase at-risk behavior.

On the other hand, when evaluating our own behavior, we point the finger to external factors. Figure 20.5 illustrates this bias in a context many readers can relate to from personal experience. This should make us stop and realize the many external variables that can be observed and often changed to increase everyone's safety-related behavior and reduce injuries throughout a culture.

> *Principle 31: When succeeding, people over attribute internal factors, but when failing, people over attribute external factors.*

This research-based principle is referred to as the "self-serving bias" (see Chapter 6) and is sure to warp injury analyses formerly called "investigations" (Chapter 9). Placing blame for a mistake on outside variables is just a basic defense to protect one's self-esteem. In most organizations, even a minor injury is perceived as a failure. As a result, the victim is sure to avoid discussing inside, person factors contributing to the mishap.

> *Principle 32: People feel more personal control when working to achieve success than when working to avoid failure.*

The sense of having control over life events is one of the most important person states contributing to our successes and failures. When we feel in control, we are more motivated and work harder to succeed. We are also more likely to accept failure as something we can change. Thus, the value of increasing people's sense of personal control over safety is obvious.

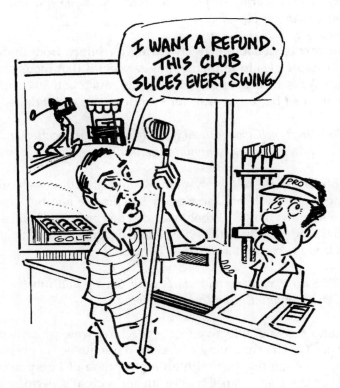

Figure 20.5 It feels better to project our imperfections on outside factors.

Principle 33: Stressors lead to positive stress or negative distress depending on appraisal of personal control.

When we believe we can do things to reduce our stressors — work demands, interpersonal conflict, boredom — we are more motivated to take control. As discussed in Chapter 6, this is positive stress, an internal person state not nearly as detrimental to safety as distress. We feel distress when we believe there is little we can do about current stressors. This state can lead to frustration, exhaustion, burnout, and dangerous behavior.

Principle 34: In a Total Safety Culture everyone goes beyond the call of duty for the safety of themselves and others — they actively care.

Here, we have a primary theme of this book. While behavior-based psychology provides methods and techniques to improve the human dynamics of safety, principles from person-based psychology need to be considered to assure the behavior-based tools are used. The ultimate aim is to integrate behavior-based and person-based psychology so everyone participates in efforts to achieve a Total Safety Culture. In the ideal culture, everyone actively cares for the safety and health of others.

Principle 35: Actively caring should be planned and purposeful and focus on the environment, person, or behavior.

Part 5 of this text is all about actively caring for safety, from understanding why people resist it (Chapter 12) to implementing strategies that increase it (Chapter 14). We need to plan ways to enable and nurture as much actively caring behavior as possible, rather than sit back and wait for "random acts of kindness."

Principle 36: Direct, behavior-focused actively caring is proactive and most challenging and requires effective communication skills.

Some acts of caring are relatively painless and effortless — contributing to a charity, sending a get-well card, or actively listening to another person's problems. Telling someone how to change his behavior can be confrontational and challenging, especially when it's direct. This is the type of active caring we are most likely to avoid, which is unfortunate because it's the most beneficial.

Principle 37: Safety coaching that starts with Caring and involves Observing, Analyzing, and Communicating leads to Helping.

The basic components of effective safety coaching were presented in Chapter 12, with each letter of COACH signifying a label for the sequence of events in the process. The coaching process should start with an atmosphere of interpersonal Caring and an agreement that the coach can Observe an individual's performance, preferably with a behavioral checklist. Then, the coach Analyzes the observations from a fact-finding, system-level perspective. Subsequently, the results are Communicated in a one-on-one actively caring conversation, with the sole purpose to Help another individual reduce the possibility of personal injury.

Principle 38: Actively caring can be increased indirectly with procedures that enhance self-esteem, belonging, and empowerment.

This principle reflects one of the most innovative and important theories presented in this book (Chapter 15). Substantial research is available to support each component of this principle. Procedures that enhance a person's sense of self-esteem ("I am valuable"), belonging ("I belong to a team"), and empowerment ("I can make a difference") make it more likely that a person will actively care for the safety or health of another person. Nourishing each of these person states leads to the actively caring belief that "We can make valuable differences."

Principle 39: Empowerment is facilitated with increases in self-efficacy, personal control, and optimism.

When people's sense of self-efficacy ("I can do it"), personal control ("I am in control"), and optimism ("I expect the best") are increased, they are more likely to feel empowered ("I can make a difference") and perform actively caring behaviors. Empowerment does not necessarily result from receiving more authority or responsibility. In order to truly feel empowered, people need to perceive they have the skills, resources, and opportunity to take on the added responsibility (self-efficacy), believe they have personal impact over their new duties (personal control), and expect the best from their efforts (optimism).

Principle 40: When people feel empowered, their safe behavior spreads to other situations and behaviors.

In a Total Safety Culture, people go beyond the call of duty for safety. This means they perform safe behaviors in various situations. They show both stimulus generalization — performing a particular safe behavior in various settings — and response generalization — performing safe behaviors related to a particular target behavior. Figure 20.6 depicts both stimulus and response generalization of actively caring.

Principle 41: Actively caring can be increased directly by educating people about factors contributing to bystander apathy.

In Chapter 16, I discussed strategies for encouraging actively caring behavior directly. This principle expresses the most basic procedure for doing this. Educating people about the barriers to helping others can remove some obstacles and increase the probability of actively caring behavior. Similarly, I have found that discussing the barriers to safe behavior can motivate people to improve safety, provided they also learn specific techniques for doing this.

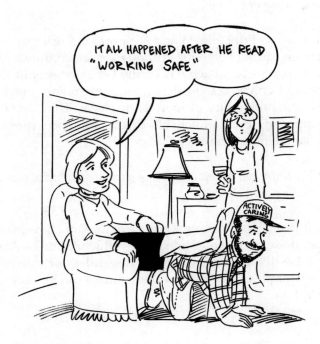

Figure 20.6 The best interventions spread their effects to other behaviors and environmental settings.

Principle 42: As the number of observers of a crisis increases, the probability of helping decreases.

This principle is probably the first barrier to actively caring behavior that should be taught. It's strange but true, and means that people can't assume someone else will intervene in a crisis. In fact, the most common excuse for not acting is something like "I thought someone else would do it," or "I didn't know it was my responsibility." This principle reflects the need to promote a norm that it's everyone's responsibility to actively care for safety.

Principle 43: Actively caring behavior is facilitated when appreciated and inhibited when unappreciated.

Making an effort to actively care directly for someone else's safety is a big step for many people and deserves genuine recognition. Then, if advice is called for to make the actively caring behavior more effective, corrective feedback should be given appropriately. Be sure to make your deposits first. All actively caring behavior is well-intentioned but not frequently practiced with the kind of feedback that shapes improvement. A negative reaction to an act of caring can be quite punishing and severely discourages a person from trying again. Consequently, much of the future of actively caring behavior is in the hands of those who receive people's attempts to actively care.

Principle 44: A positive reaction to actively caring can increase self-esteem, empowerment, and sense of belonging.

This is a follow-up to Principle 43 and supports the need to sincerely recognize occurrences of actively caring behavior. Although research in this area is lacking, it's intuitive that feeling successful at actively caring behavior should lead to more active caring. Success should enhance self-esteem, empowerment, and belonging and so, indirectly, increase the probability of more caring acts. Thus, we have the potential for a mutually supporting cycle of actively caring influence, provided the reactions to actively caring behavior are positive.

Principle 45: The universal norms of consistency and reciprocity motivate everyday behaviors, including actively caring.

These social influence norms have a powerful impact on human behavior. Sometimes, people apply these norms intentionally to influence others. At other times, these norms are activated without our awareness. Regardless of intention or awareness, behavior-change techniques derived from these norms can be very effective. The next three principles explain.

Principle 46: Once people make a commitment, they encounter internal and external pressures to think and act consistently with their position.

This is why I say you can act people into thinking differently or think people into acting differently. If people act in a certain way on the "outside," they will adjust their "inside" — including perceptions, beliefs, and attitudes — to be consistent with their behaviors. The reverse is also true, but throughout this text I have recommended targeting behavior first because it's easier to change on a large scale.

Figure 20.7 depicts a humorous scenario of rational behavior preceding the internal emotion of fear. Is this realistic? Is it reasonable to believe that this act of running from a bear will come *before* an internal person state? In fact, this is likely what happens, as predicted by the James-Lange theory of emotion. As James (1890) put it, "We feel sorry because we cry, angry because we strike, and afraid because we tremble" (page 1066).

Principle 47: The consistency norm is responsible for the impact of "foot-in-the-door."

As detailed in Chapter 16, the "foot-in-the-door" technique of social influence succeeds because of the consistency norm (Principle 46). When an individual agrees with a relatively small request, for example, to serve on a safety committee, you have your foot in the door. To be consistent, the person is more likely to agree later with a larger request, perhaps to give a safety presentation at a plant-wide meeting. Similarly, when people sign a petition or promise card that commits them to act in a certain way, say, to actively care for the safety of others, they experience pressure from the consistency norm to follow through.

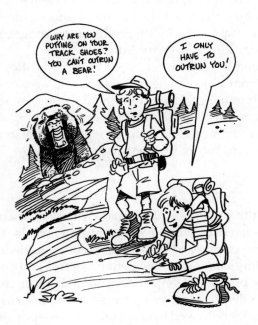

Figure 20.7 Behavior precedes emotion: we are afraid because we run.

Principle 48: The reciprocity norm is responsible for the impact of the door-in-the-face technique.

The success of the "door-in-the-face" technique depends on the reciprocity norm. If an employee shuts the door on a major request, he's more likely to be open to a lesser request. If you ask for something less imposing, costly, or inconvenient after the initial refusal, your chances of being accepted are greater than if you started with the minor request. Your willingness to withdraw the larger request sets up an obligation to reciprocate and accept the smaller request.

Principle 49: Numbers from program evaluations should be meaningful to all participants and direct and motivate intervention improvement.

The last two principles relate to the critical issue of program evaluation (Chapter 18). In safety, the total recordable injury rate (TRIR) is the most popular evaluation number used to rank companies for safety rewards. It's calculated by multiplying the number of workplace injuries by 200,000 and dividing the answer by the total person-hours worked in that time period. What an obvious example of an abstract number with little meaning! The most direct measure of ongoing safety performance comes from behavioral observations and, in Chapters 8, 12, and 18, I recommended ways to obtain meaningful feedback numbers from such process evaluation.

Principle 50: Statistical analysis often adds confusion and misunderstanding to evaluation results, thereby reducing social validity.

Complex statistics are appropriate and often necessary for research journals. If the purpose of a program evaluation is to improve a safety process, we need to provide numbers that give the most meaningful feedback to program participants — the people in the best position to improve the process.

Recall also the lesson from Chapter 5 that group statistics have minimal impact on risk perception. If your objective is to increase risk awareness and motivate safe behavior, the most influential evaluation tool you can use is actually anecdotal. The most moving feedback usually comes from the personal report of an injured employee. Therefore, the work culture needs to support reporting personal injuries, as well as discussing ways to prevent future incidents.

In conclusion

This chapter reviews the principles of human dynamics discussed throughout this book. Founded on research published in scientific journals, they enable profound understanding of the psychology of safety. Use them as guidelines to develop, implement, evaluate, and refine safety-improvement programs and you will make a positive difference in the safety of your organization, community, or culture.

Champions are needed to lead this process. Some are easy to find; others will evolve when the principles reviewed here are taught. Give potential champions opportunities to teach these principles and help develop interventions. Active participation increases both belief in the principles and the empowerment to apply them to achieve a Total Safety Culture.

There is no quick-fix to culture change. The journey is not to be without bumpy roads, forced detours, and missed turns. These principles are your map to reach an enviable destination, but be prepared to blaze new paths and traverse difficult terrain. Please do not forget to take a break now and then to appreciate journey milestones. Recognize behaviors that contribute to a successful journey.

At the end of the second Deming workshop I attended, a participant raised his hand to ask one final question. When acknowledged, he stood and walked to the nearest microphone and stated, "Dr. Deming, you have taught us many important principles to consider when designing procedures to transform a culture. But frankly, the challenge seems overwhelming. Can we really expect to make a difference in our lifetime?"

W. Edwards Deming, at age 92, replied, "That's all you've got!"

References

Bird, F. E., Jr. and Germain, G. L. (1997). *The Property Damage Accident: The Neglected Part of Safety.* Loganville, GA: Institute Publishing.

Brown, H. J., Jr. (1991). *Life's Little Instruction Book.* Nashville, TN: Rutledge Hill Press.

Bugelski, B. R. and Alimpay, D. A. (1961). The role of frequency in developing perceptual sets. *Canadian Journal of Psychology,* 5, 205–211.

Carnegie, D. (1936). *How to Win Friends and Influence People* (1981 ed.). New York: Simon & Schuster, Inc.

Cialdini, R. B. (2001). *Influence: Science and Practice* (4th ed.) New York: Harper Collins College.

Covey, S. R. (1989). *The Seven Habits of Highly Effective People: Restoring the Character Ethic.* New York: Simon & Schuster.

Daniels, A. C. (2000). *Bringing Out the Best in People* (2nd ed.). New York: McGraw-Hill.

Deming, W. E. (1985). Transformation of western style of management. *Interfaces,* 15 (3), 6.

Deming, W. E. (1986a). Drastic Changes for Western Management. Abstract for the meeting of TIMS/ORS at Gold Coast City, Australia.

Deming, W. E. (1986b). *Out of the Crisis.* Cambridge, MA: Massachusetts Institute of Technology, Center for Advanced Engineering Study.

Deming, W. E. (1991). *Quality, productivity, and competitive position.* Four-day workshop presented in Cincinnati Ohio by Quality Enhancement Seminars, Inc.

Deming, W. E. (1992). *Quality concepts to solve societal crises: Profound knowledge for psychologists.* Invited address at the Centennial Convention of the American Psychological Association, Washington, D.C.

Deming, W. E. (1993). *The New Economics for Industry, Government, Education.* Cambridge, MA: Massachusetts Institute of Technology, Center for Advanced Engineering Study.

Drebinger, J. W., Jr. (2000). *Mastering Safety Communication: Communication Skills for a Safe, Productive and Profitable Workplace* (2nd ed.). Galt, CA: Wulamoc Publishing.

Editors of Conari Press. (1993). *Random Acts of Kindness.* Emeryville, CA: Conari Press.

Frankl, V. (1962). *Man's Search for Meaning: An Introduction to Logotherapy.* Boston: Beacon Press.

Fulghum, R. (1988). *All I Really Need to Know I Learned in Kindergarten.* New York: Ivy Brooks.

Gardner, H. (1993). *Multiple Intelligences.* New York: Basic Books.

Geller, E. S. (1994). Ten principles for achieving a total safety culture. *Professional Safety,* 39 (9), 18.

Geller, E. S. (1998a). *Beyond Safety Accountability: How to Increase Personal Responsibility.* Neenah, WI: J. J. Keller & Associates.

Geller, E. S. (1998b). *Building Successful Safety Teams: Together Everyone Achieves More.* Neenah, WI: J. J. Keller & Associates.

Goleman, D. (1995). *Emotional Intelligence.* New York: Bantam Books.

Goleman, D. (1998). *Working with Emotional Intelligence.* New York: Bantam Books.

Grote, D. (1995). *Discipline without Punishment.* New York: American Management Association.

Guastello, S. J. (1993). Do we really know how well our occupational accident prevention programs work? *Safety Science,* 16, 445.

Haddon, W., Jr. (1968). The changing approach to the epidemiology, prevention, and amelioration of trauma: the transition to approaches etiologically rather than descriptively based. *American Journal of Public Health*, 58, 1431.

Hall, E. T. (1966). *The Hidden Dimension*. Garden City, NY: Doubleday.

Hansen, L. (1994). Rate your B.O.S.S.: Benchmarking organizational safety strategy. *Professional Safety*, 39(6), 37.

Heinrich, H. W., Petersen, D., and Roos, N. (1989). *Industrial Accident Prevention: A Safety Management Approach* (5th ed.). New York: McGraw-Hill.

James, W. J. (1890). *Principles of Psychology*. New York: Holt.

Langer, E. J. (1997). *The Power of Mindful Learning*. Reading, MA: Perseus Books.

Latané, B., and Darley, J. M. (1970). *The Unresponsible Bystander: Why Doesn't He Help?* New York: Appleton-Century-Crofts.

Lloyd, S. R. (1996). *Leading Teams: The Skills for Success*. West Des Moines, IA: American Media.

Mager, R. F. and Pipe, P. (1997). *Analyzing Performance Problems or You Really Oughta Wanna* (3rd. ed.). Atlanta, GA: The Center for Effective Performance.

Maslow, A. H. (1943). A Theory of Human Motivation. *Psychological Review*, 50, 370.

Milgram, S. (1963). Behavioral Studies of Obedience. *Journal of Abnormal Social Psychology*, 67, 371.

Milgram, S. (1974). *Obedience to Authority*. New York: Harper Collins.

Norman, D. A. (1988). *The Psychology of Everyday Things*. New York: Basic Books.

Parker, G. M. (ed.). (1996). *The Handbook of Best Practices for Teams* (Vol. 1). Amherst, MA: HRD Press.

Pavlov, I. P. (1927). *Conditional Reflexes*. (G. Anrep, Ed. and Trans.). London: Oxford University Press.

Peck, M. S. (1979). *The Different Drum: Community Making and Peace*. New York: Simon & Schuster.

Piliavin, J. A., Dovidio, J. F., Gaertner, S. L., and Clark, R. D., III. (1981). *Emergency Intervention*. New York: Academic Press.

Rees, F. (1997). *Teamwork from Start to Finish*. San Francisco, CA: Jossey-Bass.

Rotter, J. B. (1966). Generalized expectancies for internal versus external control of reinforcement. *Psychological Monographs*, 80(1).

Sandman, P. M. (1991). *Risk 5 Hazard + Outrage: A Formula for Effective Risk Communication*. A videotape presented to the American Industrial Hygiene Association, Environmental Communication Research Program, Cook College, Rutgers University, New Brunswick, NJ.

Seligman, M. E. P. (1975). *Helplessness: On Depression Development and Death*. San Fransisco, CA: Freeman.

Selye, H. (1974). *Stress without Distress*. Philadelphia, PA: Lippincott.

Skinner, B. F. (1938). *The Behavior of Organisms*. Acton, MA: Copley Publishing Group.

Skinner, B. F. (1974). *About Behaviorism*. New York: Alfred A. Knopf.

Skinner, B. F. (1981). Selection by consequences. *Science*, 213, 502.

Slovic, P. (1991). Beyond numbers: A broader perspective on risk perception and risk communication. In D. Mayo, and R. Hollander (Eds.), *Deceptable Evidence: Science and Values in Risk Management*. New York: Oxford.

Watson, D. L. and Tharp, R. G. (1997). *Self-Directed Behavior: Self-Modification for Personal Adjustment* (7th ed.). Pacific Grove, CA: Brooks/Cole.

Wilde, G. J. S. (1994). *Target Risk*. Toronto, Ontario, Canada: PDE Publications.

Yerkes, R. M. and Dodson, J. D. (1908). The relation of strength of stimulus to rapidity of habit formation. *Journal of Comprehensive Neurological Psychology*, 18, 459.

Index

A

ABC, see Activator-behavior-consequence model
Accident investigations, 35
Accident proneness, 6–7, 27
Accountability vs. responsibility, 123
Activator-behavior-consequence (ABC) model
    DO IT process and, 98
    human behavior and, 22, 120
    operant conditioning and, 90
    safety coaching process and, 168–169
Activators, see also Activator-behavior-consequence
    (ABC) model
    behavior influenced by, 22, 98
    intervening with, see Intervening with activators
Actively caring
    behavior-based efforts example, 194–195
    belonging and, 210–211
    categorizing behaviors, 193–194
    consequences and, 191–192, 199–201, 225
    context considerations
        definition of context, 201
        safety at work and, 202
    continuous improvement and, 191–192
    described, 191
    education and training influences, 225
    factors involved, 192–193
    hierarchy of needs, 195–196
    increasing, see Increasing actively caring
    person-based approach, see Person-based
        approach to actively caring
    psychology of
        bystander apathy, 196–197
        social responsibility norm, 198
    role in Total Safety Culture, 283–284, 285, 286
    summary, 203
"Actively Caring Thank-You Cards," 225
Active resisters, 270
Aggression and perceived control by negative
    consequences, 149
Airline Lifesaver intervention example, 135–136
Alimpay, D.A., 291
"All injuries are preventable" slogan, 44–45, 222, 281
All I Really Need to Know I Learned in Kindergarten
    (Fulghum), 143

Apathy and perceived control by negative
    consequences, 149
Arousal and performance, 69–70
"As you know" phrase, 179
At-risk behavior, see also Calculated risks
    feedback process, 106
    inadvertent rewards, 115
    motivational interventions and, 121
    reduction of, 84–85
Attitude, 44
Attributional bias
    fundamental error of, 78
    self-serving bias, 78–79, 112, 282
Authority's power over safety behavior, 48–51, 277
Autobiographical bias, 179–180
Automatic vs. controlled processing, 120
Automobile safety
    seat belt use
        Airline Lifesaver example, 135–136
        buckle-up road signs example, 136–138
        cost effectiveness, 106
        Flash for Life example, 133–135
    standards for, 27–28
Avoidance contingency, 93

B

BASIC ID, 42–44, 51–52
Batten, Joe, 27
Behavior
    factors in safety culture, 19–20
    factors in systems approach, 34
    perceived risk and, 59
    psychological dimension of, 43
Behavioral safety analysis
    behavior-based training, 118–119
    critical behavior identification, see Critical
        behaviors identification
    intervention and behavior change
        accountability vs. responsibility, 123
        flow of change, 121–122
        intervention strategies, 120–121
        types of behavior, 120
    percent safe score, 109